YOUR HEART MAINTENANCE

LIMITED EDITION

DR JOHAN JANSSEN

First edition published November 2020

Published by Red Feather Publishing

Website: www.drjanssen.com.au

Cover by Steve Barwick at All in One Book Design

Cover image by Simone Anderson, age 4

ISBN 978-0-6450105-0-3 print

ISBN 978-0-6450105-1-0 ebook

Printed in Australia

CONTENTS

INTRODUCTION

I do not know everything, but neither does the internet

Doctors, nurses, and other specialists in healthcare who read this book—out of interest, or to find mistakes😀—I am asking them to keep in mind that this book is not a scientific essay but for a broad audience with or without heart complaints. It is because of this, that I am not going into detail about more experimental treatments because they could be abandoned and not find their way into mainstream medicine. Science, after all, is not standing still. Although I try my best to follow the newest thoughts and treatment methods, it is just impossible to know all the different avenues of research or to discuss them in a book like this. I do not claim to know everything. After all, a lot of important questions regarding cardiovascular disease are still not crystallized let alone answered. And if that is the case, I will talk about it. I trust this will keep the reader from getting too frustrated and prevent spending too much time on the internet. Don't get me wrong, the worldwide web is a fantastic tool, so it is no problem to look for medical information. It is full of good texts, magnificent little videos, good drawings and nice animations about the heart, but there is a lot of rubbish in between the good stuff as well. How do you make up your mind between valid information and rubbish? A good site immediately tells you who made it, why, and if it is an independent organisation. Is it a scientific or journalistic underpinned initiative? Is the information coming from a single person or from a commercial organisation? Not that all information of institutions or companies is by definition suspect, but as a "customer" you are allowed to know from which way the wind is blowing! Another measure of quality information is that on a decent website discussing health, you find contact information in case you have questions or remarks. If names or contact material is not present or hidden, then this website is probably not for you. Websites of hospitals, governments, and health organisations are usually reliable, but they do not always use normal language, and the same holds for Wikipedia. The information you find on Wikipedia is reasonably correct and up to date—mistakes or refuted assumptions are in any case being corrected much faster than in print media—but there is a practical problem: instead of explaining difficult words or jargon, Wikipedia uses hyperlinks which transfer you to other articles which again use hyperlinks to explain things, and before you know it you are already an hour down the track and you have learned only ten new things but you still don't know what you were looking for. So, in short, don't surf the web to be healthy or prevent sickness but discuss the knowledge you get on the internet with people who know what they are talking about. One of the sites I can suggest with information about cardiovascular disease is americanheartassociation.org and The Australian Heart Foundation. They explain issues in short sentences without too many difficult words and have good illustrations and short movies.

1 CONGRATULATIONS FOR YOUR NEW ENGINE...

W ell, it is not exactly something new you are buying. You did get your heart, and it is not new because it has already been pumping for a while in your chest. Even when your very first cells started to pulsate, it was not new. In contrast to an engine from the factory, your heart, just like your blood vessels attached to it and the rest of your body, is pre-programmed with the good and less perfect genes from our parents: indeed with both genetic malfunctions and beautiful qualities. It is not only because of co-incidence or training that many talented sports people have more athletes in their family or the other way around, that you have more heart disease in one family than another. All the hearts of all the people alive at this moment have a mix of all the different traits of their parents, whose hearts carry half of the traits of all the generations before them and so on. So does every heart have the history of the whole of evolution. Notwithstanding that Mother Nature did a fantastic job. She made the best pump ever, a device that even in 2020 is not to be compared to a pump made with the most advanced materials. Just calculate what happens: with an average heartbeat of 72 beats per minute x 60 for every hour x 24, a human heart beats around 100,000 times a day.

In a year that is almost 37 million beats or 3 billion if you live for 80 years. The heart of the average 100-year-old (and there are more and more of those) has beaten 36,792,000,000 beats one after each other; amazing. No mechanical pump has that lifespan, or better, can pump that often because most other mammals who have exactly the same type of pump as we—only larger or smaller—do not live that long. A lot of mammal hearts stop after a billion beats, and this is independent of the lifespan of "the owner". A Cavia Porcellus (guinea pig) who has a heart that beats 450 times a minute, is up to the billion after a couple of years. The heart of a whale that only beats 20 times per minute reaches the billion only after 80 years. It is logical that hearts of small mammals have to beat faster. One function of the mammal heart is to keep the body temperature at a certain level and the smaller the animal the larger the square centimetre surface of the skin in relation to its volume. Compared to a bottle of fizzy drink, a two-litre bottle is not a lot bigger than a one-litre bottle but has double the volume. The larger the mammal the smaller the comparison between the body surface area and the volume, and therefore the less warmth it is losing. That is why the heart of an elephant does not have to beat as fast as that of a Cavia. People are exceptions: we have at the age of 30 approximately a billion heart beats, but on average we become a lot older, and that has to do with our lifestyle, the quality of our food, and the advances of our medical knowledge. By the way, if we think Cavia's have a fast heartbeat, what about the Colibri? During flight, its heart can beat more than one thousand times per minute and the heart of a little mouse, one of the smallest mammals in the world, even beats at 1500 beats per minute.

The animal world has more intriguing stories. Did you know that the heart of a giraffe weighs more than 11 kg, is 60 cm long, and has twice the amount of blood pressure as that compared to a human being, which is needed to have the blood pump all the way up to the brain? Did you know that an octopus has three hearts? Or that a Zebra Fish can change their heart tissue if it is damaged? That last fact is fascinating for science because mammals do not have the ability to regrow their own heart tissue. With fish, amphibia, and reptiles, the heart works quite differently as warm-blooded mammals and birds all have a heart with four chambers and a completely separated pathway for blood with oxygen and blood with less oxygen. The human heart which is 300 grams on average and one and a half fists big is pumping approximately five litres of blood around the body per minute, that is more than seven thousand litres per day or over 200 million litres per life. The pathway through which the blood is pumped is via the arteries, the veins, and all the small blood vessels, all together approximately one hundred thousand kilometres long. With the blood vessels of one human being, you can walk two-and-a-half times around the earth. And to give you an idea of how powerful this pump is working, well, try to squeeze a new tennis ball because that is approximately the power that the heart has to produce to pump the blood around.

Why does the heart not get any cramps like other muscles? I mean, if your hand is copying the pump function of the heart, your fingers have to rest after a couple of minutes already. Well, the heart has a type of arranged muscle fibres that are different to the ones from the skeletal muscles. The muscles from the heart get their nutrition and energy from so-called mitochondria, which are small structures inside the cell that produce energy from the food we are eating. The more energy centres in a cell, then the more energy is available to that cell. Skeletal muscles have approximately two percent mitochondria which is perfect for the normal activity of a human being. The heart contains approximately 3.5 billion cells and is composed out of 30 to 35% mitochondria and therefore never has to stop and rest. There is always enough energy for the next beat. Still you are to be congratulated with the engine you got, whether it is in good nick or not.

This book is for those people who have a heart without a problem as well as for people whose pump is not one hundred percent. If your heart is healthy, hopefully you can get some tips here on how to keep it healthy, and if it is not one hundred percent, I hope to be able to explain what you can do about it. One thing we cannot change (as yet) is that there will be a time when my heart and your heart will do its last beat. I think it is important that the time we have, we try to live with the least amount of problems. However, it is not all in your own hands. I discussed the fact that we have an important component of our genes there, but for the most of us it is perfectly possible to not only live to a high age but also have a great quality of life.

What was first? The heart or the heartbeat? Funnily enough, the heartbeat. During pregnancy, the heart is the first organ in an embryo to be made. The little embryo has an urgent need for oxygen and growth material to be able to grow and develop into a human being. It does get nutrients from its mother, but it has to get into all corners of the tiny embryo. Until recently we thought that the first heartbeat would be three to four weeks after conception. In the embryo a little tube-like structure is formed which grows into the heart as the embryo grows. But in 2016, people from the University of Oxford found in mice experiments that the first co-ordinated contractions occur much earlier in humans, probably at 16 days. Heart muscle cells are always contracting but not always co-ordinated. However, very soon after conception they found a small group of cells which contract in the same rhythm even before the little tube has been formed. These first beats, that stimulate the growth of the heart muscle cells stimulate the forming of the heart. No heart without the heartbeat. Maybe this new finding can help us think about new strategies to repair hearts damaged by a heart attack. So, in the eighth week of pregnancy the heart is then finally completed, and you can see it beat on an echocardiogram very well. It is tiny, and now beating about 160 times per minute. There are other important differences between this small heart and the grown-up heart and blood vessel system. The lungs of a foetus are not working as yet, the child in the womb of the mother gets the oxygen through the umbilical cord and the placenta; just as with small kids and adults the heart of the foetus has two top parts of the heart called the atria and two bottom parts of the heart, the ventricles. But the unborn child has an opening in the wall between the two atrial called the foramen ovale. Also, the artery in the lungs and the aorta are connected to each other and that is very useful for the foetus: the blood from the placenta is going through the umbilical cord to the right atrium, the right atrium will get the blood towards the right ventricle and then to the lungs, but because the lungs are not working and the blood of the placenta already has the oxygen from the mother, it is more efficient to bypass the lungs. Therefore, we need connection pieces between the atria and the big blood vessels. Those connection pieces close when the child is born and starts to breathe by itself. The blood vessel that ends in the big umbilical cord closes by itself when the umbilical cord is clamped off.

The placenta requires some explanation. This temporary organ is made during pregnancy by the embryo and foetus itself. Oxygen, nutrients, and antibodies of the mother go through the placenta into the foetus and waste products made by the embryo can be cleaned up through the same way. The changeover is done through diffusion, approximately the same way our food is diffused into the body through our gut. The blood supply system of the mother is like the one from the foetus to the placenta, but the two different blood vessels are not connected to each other, therefore it is not a problem usually if the mother and the child have a different blood group. The placenta which is connected through the umbilical cord to the unborn child, keeps out a lot of dangerous substances. Unfortunately though, alcohol, parts of cigarette smoke, some viruses, and some drugs do go past the placenta and that could be a problem for the unborn baby. After the birth, the placenta loses its function. The blood supply is cut together with the umbilical cord and the placenta is removed from the body after the child has been born. Once the child is born, its small circulation system starts. The heart of a just born baby is still beating extremely fast, but usually already some-what slower than early in pregnancy. Also, in the womb the heartbeat varies under the influence of the position of the foetus or because the mother is suffering from anxiety or an illness. From birth, the heart beats slower every month and every year. Babies older than three months have still a heart frequency around 90 to 120 beats per minute, but as the child is growing, it drops down to approximately 72 beats per minute.

2 TWO FOR THE PRICE OF ONE

Before I go into more detail about how our engine works, I would like to explain the most important parts and the construction of this fantastic machine. I will also introduce some of the most-used scientific terms, and that could be useful if you ever have to read a medical report or are in contact with a doctor who uses too much medical terminology.

Our engine looks more like a fat pear which is put on its head than the love heart you see in most cartoons from Cupid or on Valentine's day. By the way, the heart is not located in the left side of your chest or thorax, even though it is drawn there often, but in the middle of the chest just behind the breastbone or sternum. That is the place of the mediastinum, an empty space surrounded on both sides by the lung, and on the front and back side of the sternum and the spinal column. Next to the heart you will also find important pipes like the windpipe, your oesophagus, nerves, the aorta, and other big blood vessels. You will also find lymph nodes and in kids the thymus which is an important gland managing the immune system. So, the heart is situated right in the middle but a little bit more to the left than the right side behind the breastbone. In medicine we always use the words 'left' and 'right' looking from the body that we talk about. The top part of the heart is situated towards the back and to the right, so that the pointy point of the heart, called the apex, is a couple of centimetres behind the sternum and pushing into the left lung. The bottom part of the heart is resting on the diaphragm, the structure between your chest and your tummy (abdomen).

The heart consists of three layers; the outer layer is the little sac called pericardium, a strong tissue which encompasses the heart muscle. The middle layer is the heart muscle itself called the myocardium. When doctors talk about a heart attack or a myocardial infarction, they sometimes use the abbreviation MI. The inner side of the myocardium is the third layer which is called the endocardium, and this is more like the lining of a suit or a dress. It is thin and in direct contact with the blood that is being pumped through the heart. The atria and ventricles—we have two of each—are the four cavities of the heart. At the top part of the heart we find the left and right atrium. Underneath the atria, we have the left and the right chamber called the ventricles. The atria suck the blood into the heart, the ventricles pump it out again. You can also divide the heart standing upright in two sides, the right side and the left side. It is even more astounding that we see the heart as one organ, but really there are two organs who are grown together but manage different circuits. The atrium and the ventricle on the right side are completely separated from the left side through a wall. The right side takes care of the small circulation, the left side for the big circulation. The separation between the left and the right side is necessary because we would like to keep the blood with low oxygen content separated from the blood with a high oxygen content. The low oxygen content blood supply is being pumped from the right heart to the lungs to get some oxygen and then put into the left side of the heart, which takes care that the whole body gets oxygen and fuel.

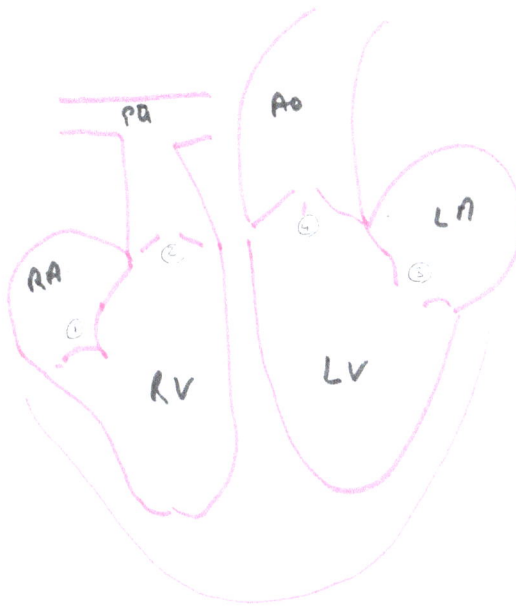

1. Schematic drawing of the right ventricle (RV), left ventricle (LV), left and right atrium (LA & RA), aorta (Ao) and pulmonary artery (PA). 1=tricuspid valve, 2=pulmonary valve, 3=mitral valve, 4=aortic valve. See also on YouTube under 'heart anatomy'.

The heart is a crossroad of blood vessels. There are two kinds of blood vessels, the veins and the arteries. The veins bring the blood to the heart, the arteries take the blood away from the heart. Sometimes you hear people talking about their veins are carrying blood without oxygen and arteries carrying blood with a lot of oxygen, but that isn't always true. We will talk about that in a second. In pictures, we find both sides of the heart and both circulations often coloured in red and blue, red is for the oxygen rich and blue for the oxygen poor. Oxygen rich blood is indeed very bright red; the colour comes from the haemoglobulin. It is a red protein that transports oxygen and CO_2 through the blood. In every red blood cell, there are approximately two hundred and seventy million haemoglobulin molecules which carry a maximum of four oxygen and four CO_2 molecules every time. Haemoglobulin also contains iron and that is why blood has a metal taste. Less oxygenated blood is not really blue but is darker red. Because veins sometimes look blue through your skin the vein blood looks blue, and that is the reason why we decided to make the veins and the right side of the heart blue and the left red. It is not that blue blood is impossible from a biological point of view; there are some crabs and octopus who have blue blood, and that is because these animals do not use haemoglobulin but haemocyanin for their oxygen transport. There are also some worms who have pink blood, some salamanders have green blood, and ice fish have white blood. Why they say that the Count's and Duchesses of this world have blue blood, we don't know. Perhaps it was because the blue pigment was difficult to find in nature for which reason it became a status symbol. Maybe you could see through the fair skin of the nobles' blue veins, and they were fair skinned because they didn't have to work in the sun. Because the arteries are prone to withstand large changes in pressure, they are very strong and elastic. The biggest artery is the aorta, 2 x 3cm in diameter, which originates from the left ventricle and after five or six centimetres makes a sharp turn to the left going down through your chest into your tummy and then to the legs. At the beginning of the aorta we find the coronary arteries, the right and the left one. These arteries give the heart its oxygen and in the curve of the aorta are the blood vessels that supply the head and the arms. The downward part of the aorta goes through the chest and the abdomen with side branches to all organs, the legs and the other parts of the body.

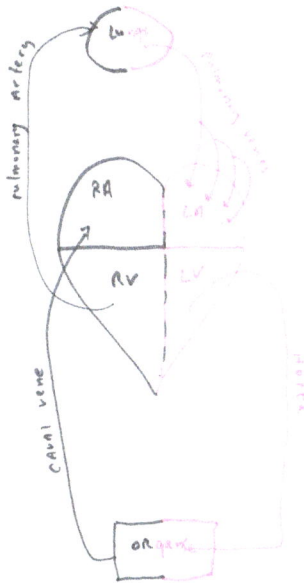

2. Schematic drawing of our circulation (see text). In black (left) the less oxygenated blood flow, in red (right) the oxygenated blood flow.

When the arteries become smaller and smaller, we call them arterials. They transport the blood to the organs and tissues, and they change into very tiny blood vessels called capillaries. The capillaries are much thinner than a hair. It is through these little blood vessels that the fuel and oxygen is delivered to cells in the tissues and organs. The little blood vessels then take on the CO_2 and other rubbish from the cells in the tissue and then come together in venules which congregate in bigger veins. In the veins, the blood travels back to the heart under low pressure and because the veins have lower pressures, they are thinner and not as strong and elastic as the arteries. They are often closer to the surface of the body and have little valves which make sure that the venous blood under the influence of gravity is not in your boots all the time. The larger veins are all collected in two big ones, one from the top part of the body and one from the bottom part of the body. Those two are then connected to the right atrium and this whole system is called the larger circulation.

The smaller circulation also starts from the heart, from the right ventricle we have the pulmonary artery which when it leaves the heart is immediately separated into the right and the left pulmonary artery in order to supply your right and left lung. The lung capillaries then come into long venules which carry the oxygen rich blood through the lung arteries back to the heart, this time to the left atrium. So this is the only time that the veins carry oxygen rich blood. In the atria we have four big veins, two on the left and two on the right. In the right atrium those are the top and the bottom hollow vein. The top one is called the vena cava superior which brings the oxygen-poor blood from the head and the top part of the body to the heart. The bottom called the vena cava inferior brings oxygen-poor blood from the bottom part of the body. In the left atrium we have also two big veins—the lung veins or pulmonary veins, one from each lung. Now the blood is in the atria and it has to get into the ventricles. That happens through valves. They make sure that the blood is only going from the atrium to the ventricles and not the other way around. There is also a valve between the ventricles and the arteries so that the blood can only go from the ventricles to the arteries when the ventricles are contracting.

How does the blood get through the heart?

Let's follow the route that the blood takes when it goes through the heart. We will start in the top part of the heart in the right atrium when low oxygen content blood from the body arrives. This is the start of the small circulation system. As soon as the right atrium is contracting, the blood is pumped into the right ventricle. It passes the valve with three leaflets or the tricuspid valve. *Tri* means three and *cuspis* is Latin for a pointy lobe because this valve has three little leaves. Just as in the other heart valves, the tricuspid valve can open in one direction. From the right ventricle the oxygen-low blood streams through the valve that separates the ventricle from the lungs —called the pulmonic valve—and then it is pumped into the lungs to get the oxygen. The lung arteries are the only arteries that carry oxygen-less blood. The then oxygenated blood from the small circulation arrives back in the heart into the left atrium. When the atrium contracts the blood, it flows into the left ventricle through a two-leaflet valve called the mitral valve. 'Mitre' is a headpiece of a bishop, which looks pointy like the valve. The left ventricle then contracts, and the oxygenated blood goes through the aortic valve into the aorta. The aortic valve has three leaflets. Of all the four chambers of the heart, the left ventricle must work the hardest. This left ventricle has to pump the oxygenated blood all the way through the smallest part of your body like your toe or the top of your head, that is why the muscle around the left ventricle is the thickest part, around 12mm.

We looked at the way the blood travels through the heart as if each of the four cavities is contracting by itself, but that is not true. Actually, it contracts two by two. First both the atria are contracting together and then the ventricles do the same, so at the same moment we have oxygen-poor blood and oxygen-rich blood sucked into the heart and at the same time we pump the oxygen-rich and oxygen-poor blood out of the heart. To be perfectly correct, the atria are not exactly pumping together and that is because the start of the heartbeat is situated at the top part of the right atrium so that the right atrium is a fraction of a second earlier in contraction than the left atrium. The ventricles however contract perfectly synchronous, however, they start at exactly the same time but not as long as each other, the right ventricle relaxes just a little bit earlier than the left ventricle. The left ventricle pumps the blood into the body which has more resistance, hence it has to work just a little bit longer for each heartbeat, and so takes a slightly more time compared to the right.

3 FUEL FOR THE ENGINE ITSELF

The heart muscle itself also needs oxygen of course. It is of interest that the heart muscle itself does not get too much oxygen out of the blood it is pumping around. The majority of the oxygen is supplied by two arteries that start out of the root of the aorta very close to the heart and are full of oxygen. These are the so-called coronary arteries. They are called coronary arteries because they are like a crown around the outside of the heart where they cannot be squeezed by the heart muscle when it is contracting. You have a right and a left coronary artery. The left one has two big branches; one is a descending branch on the front and another one that circles around the heart. They are called the 'left anterior descending' or LAD and the circumflex artery. The left coronary artery with its two big branches supplies most humans the largest part of the heart muscle, approximately 65%, while the right coronary artery takes care of the remaining 35%. Both coronary arteries have many small branches that find their way inside the heart muscle itself and become very tiny blood vessels supplying the heart cells (myocytes) with oxygen and nutrients. The pattern of distribution of the coronary arteries is, by the way, very different in different people; some people have only one coronary artery, others, approximately 4% of the population have three. The third coronary artery is then on the back side of the heart. These are differences that one is born with—so-called congenital differences. But even in people with "normal distribution" of the coronary arteries, there are many differences in how exactly the arteries go around and inside the heart muscle and that fact makes it only more exciting for us Cardiologists when we have to try to open up a narrowing in one of those coronary arteries. We have to find the right way to get there in the first place. There is yet another difference; in some people there is a connection between the main coronary arteries which can alleviate the lack of blood supply if there is a narrowing. We call those 'collateral circulation'. However, we do all have coronary veins which transport the less oxygenated blood when the heart is finished with the oxygenated blood away from the heart back into the caval vein, but those usually do not cause any problems hence you don't read about it much.

You have two types of heart cells. You have the muscle cells or the cardiomyocytes, and you have pacemaker cells. The cardiomyocytes form the atria and the ventricles and are flexible enough to contract, then relax and contract again which means that the heart can pump. Cardiac myocytes get larger when the heart grows from a child's heart to an adult heart, but also under the influence of intensive sports and some heart disease. Recent investigations did show that a part of the cardiac myocytes is replaced later on in life just like other cells, but in general heart cells do stop multiplying pretty quickly. A sports heart does not have more but only bigger myocytes. Because heart cells have a tendency to multiply less, you will never have heard of heart cancer. The cancer does exist but is very rare. Usually it is related to spreading of other cancers that attack the heart muscle.

The pacemaker cells can make electrical impulses and transmit them, but they can also react on electrical signals from the brain. They not only have quite a different function than the cardiac myocytes, but they also look different—larger and lighter in colour. Our engine, the heart, continues to do its job because its cells are electrically stimulated to contract. That stimulus is made by the heart itself in the so-called 'sinus node'. The sinus node is a group of pacemaker cells placed on a banana-like area in the top part of the wall of the right atrium. The sinus node cells are firing their electrical activity faster than all the other pacemaker cells and override them, so to speak. If the sinus node did not work properly, then the heart is still beating but much slower. The sinus node is the real stimulator of the heart. It dominates and makes the normal rhythm. The little electrical current it produces goes very fast at 58 hundredths of a second through an electricity system throughout the heart. Firstly, the atria contract and after that the ventricles. In an adult at rest that happens an average of 72 times per minute, but the brain and more particularly the hypothalamus, can increase that frequency. The hypothalamus is a very important zone in the brain which apart from the heartbeat, can also influence the blood pressure, hunger, thirst, sleeping and waking rhythm, body temperature, and sexual excitement. If you do sports, then the hypothalamus makes your heart beat faster, but at rest or during normal circumstances the sinus node cells itself produce around 70 beats per minute. You will notice that if you take a beating heart out of a mammal; it still continues to beat for a little while. In a human heart that will take only a few seconds, but in 2013 an American Cardiac Surgeon put images of an explanted heart on You Tube. The patient received a heart transplant, and that heart was beating for more than 25 minutes on its own! A beating heart that is being explanted will stop after some time because it doesn't get any glyconutrients or oxygen, not because it is not connected to the nervous system. Thus, the stimulation centre that makes the heart beat is situated in the heart itself.

The electrical activity of the sinus node will be propagated through the heart like little domino tiles that fall over and activate all the cells.

Between the atrium and the ventricle, however, is an isolating layer where the electricity cannot pass and that is why the atria and the ventricles do not contract together, not yet. There is one little spot, the so-called atrioventricular node (AV), located between the atria and the ventricle that conducts the electrical activity from the sinus node down to the ventricles. That node is situated in the left lower part of the right atrium on the border between the left atrium and the tissue in between both atria and ventricles. It is only for a moment—a couple of hundredths of a second—that the electrical activity of the sinus node is held in the AV node, and that allows the atria to contract and pump the blood physically into the ventricles before the ventricles contract. The AV node then passes the electrical activity via the septum which is the differentiation between the left and the right ventricle, and in there we find the very specialised electrical system that is called the "bundle of His". That bundle takes the electrical impulse along three bundles to the apex of the heart which is on the bottom part of the heart. From there, there are so-called "Purkinje fibres" going up that organise the electrical activity to go to all the cells in the ventricles, the reason why they can synchronously contract.

The weird names of those vessels are related to the 19th century scientist, the Swiss Wilhelm His Jnr and the Czech Jan Evangelista Purkinje who found those particular electrical fibres. The electrical system makes the heart pump in the right order and in the right rhythm. First the atria and then the ventricles, and just long enough for the double pump to get enough blood into the heart and out of the heart. If the system is out of synch you have a heart rhythm problem, and your heart is not working properly. Sometimes humans can die from these, but most abnormalities of the heart rhythm are pretty innocent or can be treated with medication, a pacemaker, or surgery.

THE ECG

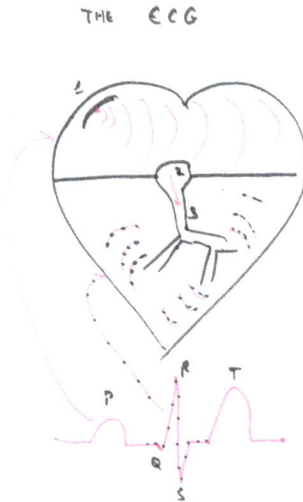

3. Schematic drawing of the electricity system of the heart.
1=sinus node, 2=AV node, 3=his bundle and bundle branches
(see text). The electrical activity of the heart can be measured by
means of a surface electrocardiogram (ECG or EKG). The
electrical impulse going over the top part of the heart, both atria, is
depicted on the ECG as a P wave. The time it takes for the
electrical activity to travel from the sinus node into the AV node
is called the PR interval. The QRS complex is the graphical
representation of the electrical impulse going over both ventricles.
The T wave is the graphical representation when the heart is 'at
rest', so that it can be reactivated during the next heartbeat. See
also YouTube 'heartbeat'.

What you hear is the closing of the heart valves

The moment when the left and the right ventricle contract we call it
the "systole". Perhaps you have heard of systolic blood pressure? That
is the pressure in the ventricles which causes the mitral and the
tricuspid valve to close so that no blood can be pumped back into the
left and right atria and it opens the aortic and pulmonary valve so
that the blood can travel from the heart into the pulmonary artery

and into the aorta. After this, the whole heart can relax for a moment, that relaxing phase is called the "diastole", the resting phase of the heart cycle where the atria and ventricles are being filled with blood. At the end of the diastole, the atria contract again, more blood is being pumped in the ventricles, they come under pressure, the valve between the atrium and ventricles are pushed shut, and you can hear the sound of the closing valves if you listen with your ear or a stethoscope on the chest. As a matter of fact, it is not the valves that you hear but the turbulence of the blood as a consequence of this process. The second heart tone originates from the two other valves who close just after the systole.

Feel your pulse. As you can hear your heart beat you can also feel it. You can feel your radial pulse—the one on your inner wrist—but apart from that there are also quite a few other places where you can feel the heartbeat, like in your neck, in your groin, in your ankles, and on your temple. A lot of people have problems finding the pulse, they feel much too much and / or press too hard in the middle of the pulse between the muscles. If you just put your hand with the palms upside and you feel with your index and middle finger of the other hand softly on the wrist you will most likely feel it. In babies up to two years you can also very carefully feel the heartbeat at the fontanelle on top of the head, you can even see the heartbeat there.

Men's and women's hearts

Considering the way the electricity or the pump are built, women's hearts are mostly the same as men's hearts. However, doctors have recently recognised differences between the two. We knew for quite some time that the heart of women beats a little bit faster and with a little bit smaller volume. The mean heart volume of a man is around 770cc while for a woman 560cc. Women also have smaller coronary arteries, and the inside of the coronary arteries are more sensitive to hormones and stress. It is important to know that some diseases of the heart in women present differently and have a different cause than in men. For instance, women have often more diffuse narrowing's in the coronary arteries whilst in men they are more in the same fixed places and often therefore also more troublesome. We have known for a couple of years that in women there are different immune cells and inflammation cells active when there is an obstruction in the coronary arteries as compared to men. A lot of people still think that heart disease is a man's disease, which is not correct. Every year more women than men die from heart disease. Also, the symptoms of a heart attack can be different between both genders. If men with a significant narrowing in the coronary arteries go to the doctor they complain often about a pressing pain on the chest, while women talk about having more fatigue, shortness of breath, or pain in the back. These are vaguer complaints which are often confused with their periods or menopause. This is unfortunate and also dangerous!

Three different disciplines

We can talk a lot more about the way the heart has been built and how it works. The heart is an amazing organ. What we just discussed however is enough to have an idea about how a normal healthy heart works so we can discuss now what happens if we have a defect or a mishap of the heart. Remember that the heart is a very strong muscle pump, very well-tuned, but even the best piece of equipment goes down the drain if you don't look after it, if you let it rust, or if you don't read the instructions! What I think is very interesting is the play between the three technical aspects of the heart: the mechanics, the plumbing, and the electricity. You have the mechanical system of the heart as a double pump which is pumping the blood through your body. You have the plumbing of the coronary arteries, the very complicated, very large tubing system of arteries and veins, and then we have the electricity which goes through the heart cells and produces the electricity to make the heart contract. The mechanics, plumbing, and electricity of the heart are constantly influencing each other. If the tubes get blocked, the mechanics start sputtering, and the electricity is staggered, if there is a leaking valve or there is a problem with the cardiac myocytes and the electrical impulses, then the pump does not work anymore and that is what we are going to discuss next.

4   MALFUNCTION, DEFECTS AND ALERT SIGNS

Heart and vascular disease

Cardiovascular disease is the most important cause of death in humans. Every year around the world almost 80 million people die because of cardiovascular disease. Cardiovascular diseases (CVD) are approximately one third of all causes of death and 80% of those deaths are due to heart attacks and strokes. The number one cause of death is not malaria, not tuberculosis, not another infectious disease, but a group of non-transmittable diseases like heart and blood vessel disease, followed by cancer (almost 9 million deaths per year), breathing /respiratory problems (almost 4 million a year), and diabetes (approximately 1.5 million a year). These non-communicable diseases are together the cause of 80% (40 million of all deaths), even though they do not get as much coverage in the news than famine or pandemics like COVID-19. The reason cardiovascular disease has taken so many people and made them ill or killed them is because of the combination of genetic factors and the way we live: the wrong food, smoking, and not enough exercise/movement. Also, outside the western world CVD's are getting more and more preva-lent. Together with our fast food and soft drink culture, we have introduced with our "well-to-do" lifestyle , problems as obesity, diabetes and coronary artery disease. Another reason for the high number of casualties caused by cardiovascular disease is that we are on average getting older and of course you have to die of something. Often it is by cancer or a cardiovascular disease.

Cardiovascular diseases are classically divided into hereditary and acquired disease. Hereditary is one you are born with, whereas acquired conditions occur sometime in your life because of an infec-tion, a less than optimal lifestyle, accidents, etc. It could also be a combination, a disease which you have because of your genetic predisposition but which only becomes evident because of non-hereditary factors like smoking. The difference between those two is not always that clear or relevant. I think it is more practical to focus on the most important mechanisms which according to many scien-tists, are on the basis of the cardiovascular disease spectrum. After that we will discuss the most common diseases and demonstrate how they are related to each other.

What are some common misunderstandings?

Before you go and surf the internet it is important to realise some misunderstandings. These misunderstandings are caused because different definitions are not always being used correctly and are not always synonymous, for instance a heart attack or a heart infarction or a stopping heart, failing heart, broken heart, flat line, asystole, sudden death, cardiac death, and so forth. In the media and by many people these terms are indiscriminately used, and people think that they are more or less the same.

A heart attack or an infarct are synonymous for what we call in cardi-ology a "myocardial infarction": a problem in a coronary artery causing the blood supply to a part of the heart muscle to cease, but as a result that part of the heart muscle is dying. Because of the myocardial infarct the pump function of the heart can be impaired but that is not always the case. Myocardial infarcts more often do not cause death.

Heart standstill or the heart stopped? That is a misleading term because the heart does not stand still when we talk about a standstill or stopping heart. The most common cause of the heart stopping is ventricular fibrillation, when the rhythm is going very fast, is chaotic, and superficial in the ventricles. In this situation there is still electrical activity in the heart, and it is moving very fast. But there is no contraction so there is no pump function, and the blood is not being pushed around. The heart is not functioning. Ventricular fibrillation is life threatening and without immediate help it can lead to death within several minutes. It can only be treated with electrical shock. This electrical shock is called defibrillation. If you have ventricular fibrillation outside the hospital and do not receive immediate reanimation with cardiac massage and defibrillation, then the risk that you will die is higher than 90%.

Heart failure is different to a heart attack or a standstill. You read once in a while that a young athlete died because of heart failure but there is usually a more acute problem like an arrhythmia or an aneurysm that burst. Heart failure is an aging process where the heart is less and less able to pump enough blood around. With every contraction, a healthy heart can pump almost 75% of the blood in the left ventricle to the aorta, a failing heart eventually can only push a little bit of blood and in the end nothing at all.

A dissection is a rupture of the aorta, our largest artery, caused by a trauma, accident, or where it has burst in a weak spot. If the tear is big you lose a lot of blood immediately and there is no circulation. Without immediate specialised help your chances of survival are zero.

"Flatline" is something most people recognise from hospital series on television. You will see on the heart monitor how the little peaks on the ECG and the peep sounds are being disrupted and changed into a straight line with a very long peep sound. That can mean two things —the device is not working, or we do not recognise any electrical heart activity. In our jargon we call that asystole. In the past you saw on television that they would jump on the patient and would give electrical shocks and so forth, but it doesn't happen anymore. The shocks are delivered with a defibrillator. This device works because it stops the irregularity of the electricity by putting the electrical activity in all heart muscle cells at the same time on zero. You could argue that a defibrillator actually causes a short asystole before the heart regains its normal heartbeat. It is what you could call a heart reset. With a flatline there is nothing thrilling any more so there is nothing to de-thrill. When you have a flatline you can only try to get the heart going again with medication, usually we use Epinephrine.

With heart deaths or sudden deaths, we usually mean the sudden but unexpected demise of a person by an unknown or not so clear heart problem. If you don't know the underlying problem of the now not working pump or if you don't need to because the death is the most important issue, then you talk usually about sudden cardiac death.

Another misunderstanding which we find regularly has to do with the different type of doctors who look for cardiovascular disease and/or treat cardiovascular disease. Sometimes we talk about heart specialists, then we talk about Cardiologists, heart surgeons, cardiac surgeons, vascular surgeons. I make it clear I am a Cardiologist or heart specialist—that is the same thing. A Cardiologist is a specialist in diseases of the heart. Some Cardiologists have specialised in their particular field even further, for instance in the genetic aspects of heart disease or specifically in heart disease in children. I was trained as a general heart specialist and then subspecialised in the rhythm of the heart, cardiac arrhythmias, and later as an Interventional Cardiologist that solves problems of the blood supply of the heart with a balloon or stenting—I am neither a cardiac surgeon nor a vascular surgeon, but that doesn't mean that I don't do any interventions. So now we have discussed what different people are doing, we can talk about the diseases.

5   HIGH BLOOD PRESSURE

1.7 billion people with high blood pressure (hypertension)

High blood pressure or hypertension is something that happens if your blood is pushing too forcefully against the inner side of your arteries. 40% of all people over 25 years of age are in that situation according to the World Health Organisation. With a total humanity of 7.4 billion people of which almost 60% is older than 25 years of age, we are talking about 1.7 billion high blood pressure patients and at least one billion does not know that they have the problem. Those people that do know about the problem work on it too little too late. The figures are idiotic, they are almost too large to comprehend. These figures of hypertension show it is the most common and the most under recognised disease in the world despite the fact that we are taking an enormous amount of tablets every day to keep this problem under control. In Australia, one in four tablets people are taking is a drug designed to lower blood pressure. It is the most common drug used in Australia. Because of the elderly population and bad lifestyle habits, more and more people are suffering from hypertension: 20 years ago, maybe 25% of our population had high blood pressure, today more than one third.

We all live in a yellow …

What is the problem of high blood pressure? Do we have to deal with a mistake in our construction? Are we using our body wrongly? If you use a device or an instrument wrongly then the guarantee is void. And part of the explanation is that high blood pressure—not the disease in itself but the risk factor to get more diseases—is behaving like a submarine. Most medical problems declare themselves because of symptoms, but there are also diseases which can stay unrecognised without any symptoms for a long, long time before they surface and cause the problem. It often happens that for years people don't know that they have high blood pressure because the symptoms are so minimal and occur so slowly that they are not recognised, or just because you get used to it, like a frog in a pan with water that heats up slowly—he won't jump out. Osteoporosis and diabetes are examples of submarine diseases or silent killers, like colon cancer, HIV infection (that virus has an incubation period of ten years!) and … high blood pressure.

How do you measure blood pressure? The upper pressure or systolic pressure is the pressure in the arteries when the left heart is contracting and pushing the blood into the aorta. The resting pressure or diastolic pressure is the pressure when the heart relaxes and is being refilled with blood. In general, the resting pressure, the diastolic pressure, is approximately half the value of the systolic pressure plus two. You are being told that your blood pressure is 120/80 or, not as good, 160/100. Measuring the blood pressure is usually the first thing your GP does for you when you come for a consultation. How actually measuring the blood pressure works is something we will come back to later.

How high is too high?

Some time ago the norms for blood pressure were not that strict. In those days one thought that the systolic blood pressure would increase by age plus ten, plus one per ten years of age, so for somebody aged 40 with a blood pressure of 140 would be acceptable, but for somebody that was 80-years of age, 180 is much more dangerous. In today's world even small increases in blood pressure are being frowned upon and often treated. There is no clear scientific agreement that states which measurement of blood pressure increases your risk of losing your health. There is an international agreement among physicians and doctors that a blood pressure of 120/80 is ideal and high blood pressure, hypertension, starts at a blood pressure higher than 140 or a diastolic pressure higher than 90. However, there are exceptions. For some people with diabetes or a kidney problem the limits are lower—130/80. With babies, the normal blood pressure is 80/60 and when they are growing up their normal values will increase. It might be true that high blood pressure is often unrecognised but sometimes the diagnosis is also made too fast. After all, your blood pressure varies, it changes from minute to minute, from hour to hour, and day to day. It can also peak under the influence of emotion, stress, or physical exertion. These are temporary triggers of a rise in blood pressure but no real signs of hypertension. That diagnosis is only there if you have had multiple measures that confirm that your blood pressure is too high all the time. Before a blood pressure measurement, a patient should not smoke and should not drink coffee, otherwise you can have a false positive result. Blood pressure is best measured several times in the same arm and with a couple of minutes in between, then you take the average of all the measurements.

Is your blood pressure only a little bit up? Then it is better to measure the blood pressure several times, perhaps three times in the next couple of months to make sure the blood pressure really is too high.

At night your blood pressure should have a little dip of perhaps 10 to 20% lower than the average during the day. If that is not the case, you suffer from non-dipping and you have a considerable high risk of the development of cardiovascular disease. A 24-hour blood pressure measurement done with a special little device can bring this to light.

When do you have to go to a doctor?

Even when you have no symptoms, it is sensible to see a doctor from the age of 35 at least every five years to have your blood pressure checked. But as it is very easy to measure blood pressure, it is a good habit to have it done every time you see your GP—especially when you are a smoker, older than 50, known to have high blood pressure, carry too much weight, or have high cholesterol in your family.

Causes

Often, we talk about primary, idiopathic, or essential hypertension. All fancy words which mean that we don't know. In 95% of patients the doctor cannot explain why high blood pressure would occur, and he or she has to deal with a myriad of genetics, lifestyle habits, age etc. We know that the blood pressure gets higher as people get older and their arteries are less elastic, less pliable, because this problem especially occurs in the big blood vessels. Before the age of 30 years only 1 to 2% of humans have high blood pressure. In people in the population over 60-years of age that is 60%. The systolic pressure in particular rises. The diastolic pressure often drops after the age of 60, and if you are over 80 you also see that your systolic pressure drops again. Not only is age important, but also your genes, your race, and your gender are of importance. If your mum or dad have high blood pressure, then you too have a high risk of having high blood pressure. High blood pressure is also more common in black people than Caucasians, and more often in men than in women, even though that turns around with age—over the age of 60 more women have hypertension compared to men and that has to do with menopause. Sometimes hypertension is caused by another illness. It can for instance be related to kidney disease; narrowing in a kidney artery can cause high blood pressure. You can get high blood pressure when your adrenal glands on top of your kidneys make too many hormones, also a low functioning thyroid and obstructive sleep apnoea can make blood pressure go up. In children and young adults, it is sometimes because of a narrowing in the aorta and pregnant women can have a problem with pre-eclampsia.

It is also possible that some medications can cause high blood pressure. There is anecdotal evidence that the oral anticonception tablet could cause high blood pressure although nowadays with modern tablets, that is much rarer. And what about food and lifestyle you ask? Too much salt does play a role, especially if at the same time you do not get enough potassium, causing the smooth muscle of the arteries to contract more forcefully together. Alcohol is an important factor. According to science one in seven cases of high blood pressure is caused by the use of alcohol. To be heavy or have a BMI of more than 25 also increases your risk of high blood pressure and, even more important, if your tummy circumference is more than 80cm for women and more than 94 for men you have a significant risk for development of hypertension. Other risk factors are a sedentary life and, remarkably, air pollution and noise. That last item was shown in a study done with 40,000 Europeans over a long period. The conclusion was that in polluted areas there is more risk of hypertension as a result of the pollution and noise. People who live in busy streets have 6% more risk of having hypertension, 90% of Europeans are exposed to air pollution above the norms of the World Health Organisation and in 2012 that caused 482,000 premature deaths caused by cardiovascular disease and lung disease.

What happens? The arteries really suffer from the forceful pumping of the blood by the heart and are therefore prone to the results of this high pressure. In principle, we should always talk about arterial hypertension, but we usually only call it hypertension. Normal healthy arteries have a very smooth elastic inner wall where the blood smoothly streams, and the wall can manage different pressures easily without getting rigid or floppy. When one has hypertension, the blood streams with far too much force through these arteries. You don't feel anything, but the high pressure damages the wall of the arteries. If the pressure is there every time, then the wall of the artery gets very rough and is not smooth anymore. On the rough places fats and little calcified particles can stick and cause atherosclerosis. Atherosclerosis makes your arteries narrower and stiffer and that in the end will obstruct blood flow. This particular process can go on for tens of years before it troubles you. In hypertension, the wall of the blood vessel cannot only be damaged and get obstructed with athero-sclerotic plaque, but it can also rupture like a tyre. It is this mecha-nism that causes hypertension to be a risk factor for bleeding in the brain which is caused by a ruptured artery in the brain.

Another result of high blood pressure is that your heart has to pump stronger and harder because the stiffened arteries have more resis-tance to the blood flow. How bad hypertension is for an individual also depends on the other risk factors. Hypertension is not neces-sarily a big problem if all the other factors are okay. If you have a slim female of 40 years of age who does not smoke, has no diabetes, eats healthy, and has a couple of hours a week doing sports and if her blood pressure is too high, then it is much less of a problem than for an obese man of 55 who has a sedentary lifestyle, drinks a lot of beer and soft drinks and smokes a packet of cigarettes. The man has a significantly higher risk of developing heart disease or having a stroke or damaging his kidney. Because the heart of somebody with hyper-tension has to provide more power and has do a tougher job, the wall of the left side of the heart, the left ventricle, gets reactively thicker and stiffer, and in time will cause the heart to fail. So, hypertension can cause havoc. The phenomena increase the risk of atherosclerosis and therefore also the development of angina pectoris, myocardial infarction, stoke, and peripheral vascular disease. High blood pressure can be important in causing certain rhythm problems of the heart, especially atrial fibrillation. You are also more prone to have a bleed in the brain, especially if you were already born with a small aneurysm in your brain, and also your kidneys can be damaged and fail because high blood pressure damages the arteries in your kidneys. One in ten people who die from high blood pressure do so because of failing kidneys.

The measuring of the blood pressure and especially the knowledge and production of anti-hypertensive medication have significantly changed in medicine. Since the Greeks and until some years ago, people were healthy until proven otherwise. They only asked for a doctor if they had complaints. Since we have the ability to lower blood pressure however, more and more asymptomatic people are being seen, usually on their behalf to ask whether they are still healthy, and it is then the plight of the doctor to either give them peace of mind or give them a treatment plan for risk management. This is opening up the path for the doctor to act as a trouble shooter and to fix the person. They are the prevention specialist for those people who want to be in charge of their own health more and more. In the old days, the fire brigade would only come out if there were flames going through the roof, now they make promotional visits to install fire alarms and we are very keen as a society to prevent fire, we will not fall asleep with burning cigarettes in our hands any more. So I think that this important change in medicine is in large part thanks to the development of anti-hypertensive treatment.

6 HYPERCHOLESTEROLAEMIA AND DYSLIPIDAEMIA

My cholesterol level is too high

Perhaps this is the most common sentence that you hear when Australians are talking about their health, after of course comments on their blood pressure or body weight. What they are discussing is hypercholesterolaemia which is an abnormality where we have too much cholesterol in the blood stream because of genetics, eating too many bad fats, obesity or another disease such as diabetes or a slow thyroid. Just like hypertension (high blood pressure) hypercholesterolaemia (high cholesterol level) is a possible risk factor for the development of heart and blood vessel disease but we are not finished with this business from a scientific point of view.

What is cholesterol?

Although we talk and read and write a lot about cholesterol, not too many people actually know what cholesterol is and what cholesterol does in our body, or what the danger is of having too much cholesterol. That is not ignorance per se because the danger of too much cholesterol is something that doctors, and scientists are not sure of themselves. Cholesterol is a Greek word and means "solid gall". Gall stones are predominantly made out of cholesterol so that is probably what the Greeks had right. It is a waxy, fatty substance which is very important for our body. Cholesterol is part of the production of hormones, vitamin D, and gall bladder acids, which play an important role in digesting your food and the absorption of vitamins. Cholesterol improves the strength of cells and is also important in being permeable for other chemical substances. You find cholesterol in every cell of our body. You get approximately one third of your cholesterol in your body through your food and more specifically through the ingestion of animal derived products with saturated fats like meat, eggs, and cheese. The rest—the bulk of our cholesterol—is made by the body itself, in the liver.

LDL, HDL, and Triglycerides

Cholesterol is present in different forms in our body. The most well-known ones are LDL and HDL cholesterol. LDL is known as the so-called "bad cholesterol" and the HDL the "good cholesterol". Really there is only one kind of cholesterol but as such does not occur in the blood. Fats and water don't mix well together while water is still a main component of our blood, and cholesterol has to go through the blood with the blood to get in all tissues and cells. To make this possible the cholesterol makes certain connections with "transport proteins". Together then they form the lipoproteins—literally translated the "fat proteins". Two of those are very important, one with a low density (LDL, low density lipoprotein) and those with a high density (HDL, high density lipoproteins). A considerable amount of our cholesterol is, together with triglycerides, packaged in little LDL spheres which can be given to the blood and transported by the blood to tissues to do their work. The remainder of the LDL is then absorbed by HDL cholesterol and brought back to the liver, also using the blood as a transport carrier. The liver then gets rid of the cholesterol through the gall bladder and is discarded from the body. So far, no problem. The problems occur when you have too much cholesterol and when there is more LDL cholesterol in your blood than the HDL can get rid of. In that case LDL continues to circulate in your blood and that can get into the inner lining of your arteries. To be honest, we do not know for sure how HDL is really able to nullify the effects of the excess LDL. Most doctors and health departments think that if you have an elevated LDL in your blood, your risk of getting a heart or vascular disease (CVD) is increased, especially if your HDL levels are low.

I just talked about triglycerides which are also important. Triglyceride is a difficult name for the fats in oils and other fatty substances you are eating. These triglycerides can also deposit in your arteries. If you have both too much cholesterol and triglycerides in your blood, that is when you have dyslipidaemia which is in a way a larger issue than hypercholesterolaemia alone. If there are too many cholesterol and triglyceride molecules in your artery, then slowly the arteries might occlude and if there is also calcium inside this accumulation of fat then also you have calcified arteries.

How high should your cholesterol be when you look into your blood test?

Just as with hypertension (high blood pressure) you don't feel anything when you have a high cholesterol level. Probably 25% of humans between 35 and 70 years of age would have too much cholesterol in their blood, but to know whether you are also part of this club you have to do a blood test. If you often eat unhealthily, you smoke, drink too much alcohol, or you are obese, then it is a good idea to do that every year. Your doctor would probably then not only do your cholesterol, but also your triglycerides. The doctor would test your total cholesterol, HDL cholesterol, LDL cholesterol, and your triglycerides. To do a cholesterol test you don't have to fast, but to have a good idea about your complete metabolism of fats it is better to fast from 10pm the night before the blood test and just drink water. If you do eat, then the complete test results might change. Your total cholesterol is best underneath 5mmol/L, your LDL below 1.8, your HDL over 1, and your triglycerides below 2. If you want to know whether you have enough "protective cholesterol" then you subdivide your total cholesterol by your HDL. A result of 3.5 vs 1 would be ideal. If your blood test shows that you have a higher cholesterol, then there is still no drama. Perhaps it was a random finding. Just as your blood pressure goes up and down with life, your cholesterol also has certain variations, so when you have one test with an elevated cholesterol you would probably need more blood tests to make sure that you understand whether you do or do not have hypercholesterolaemia or dyslipidaemia.

To statin or not to statin?

What do you do when you have hypercholesterolaemia or dyslipidaemia? That is a very difficult question. Firstly, and very importantly: you don't have any influence on the majority of cholesterol being made by the body itself. Even the most stringent diet has only a limited effect on your cholesterol levels. The second problem is that scientists are not all in agreement. In 2016 there was a new and interesting analysis of 30 studies about the value of LDL cholesterol and the risk of getting sick or dying in patients over 60 years of age (British Medical Journal, June 12 2016, Ravnskov). The conclusions were remarkable. Of the 28 studies relating to a potential link between cholesterol and death, there were 12 studies that did not find a correlation and 16 which did find a correlation, but this was between low LDL(!) and death. Just the opposite of what we were expecting. Nine of the 30 studies were specifically designed to show the relationship between LDL and death by a cardiovascular disease. Seven did not find any correlation and, again, two studies showed a correlation between low LDL and a cardiac disease. You can imagine what in those days the newspapers said: "bad cholesterol is keeping you alive longer", you could read in *the Times*. There are all different comments and problems with this study published in the *British Medical Journal* because this study was bundling results of other investigations as a meta-analysis which does not really show a causality. It does however show that the last word about cholesterol has not yet been said. The same story is true for the medications that were used most often for high cholesterol management, the so-called statins. If you take a statin you are blocking a protein that your body needs to make cholesterol. The result is that very quickly you have in your tissue a lack of cholesterol. The body reacts to that to make LDL cholesterol present in the usable blood. The result is your cholesterol levels drop dramatically, usually within a couple of months in 50% of people anywhere in the world. That is much faster and a much better result than what you would ever get by healthy living and more exercise. It is therefore no wonder that statins were an absolute hit quickly in the top ten of medications. The downside of this distinction is that statins, like other medications, have side effects. One third of the people that use statins complain about painful, stiff, and tired muscles. Sometimes it is so bad that they cannot do their day to day activities. If I use a high dose of a statin myself, I can play one set of tennis and then I have to crawl off the tennis court. But you also have studies showing that if you give patients a placebo instead of a real statin you get the same complaint percentages. There have been other published side effects such as impotence, problems with your stomach, and rarely it does happen, but so-called rhabdomyolysis, a significant disease of your muscles which can also damage the liver and the kidneys and can kill. In any case, in 2012 the Food and Drug Administration which is the American TGA that looks over our food and medication intake, came with an official warning: statins according to the FDA would give you a higher risk of muscle pains, type 2 diabetes, and memory loss. The FDA also said however, the advantages of a statin as a way of reducing heart and blood vessel disease was much in favour of that as compared to the risk, but nevertheless thought it necessary to warn the users. The FDA is not giving us a warning for nothing, especially not when you know that the FDA is always under critique that it is too slow in reacting to the real world. But we need to be careful and not put our statins straight into the bin. I think it is important that if you have queries about the use of a statin you talk to your GP or Cardiologist, and if you are not sure, maybe with more than one. It is your decision and your responsibility to follow the advice of your doctor, but it is his or her responsibility to give you the best possible advice. In any case never cease your cholesterol lowering medication on your own accord, always discuss!

The controversy over the risk of cholesterol as well as statins is very popular on the internet. People that go into this matter on the internet, doctors as well as patients, get a headache within five minutes. There is a group of one hundred or so scientists who call themselves The International Network of Cholesterol Sceptics. They think that the medical world is interpreting the results of the investigations systematically in the wrong way. According to them, patients are being prescribed statins to keep the pharmacological industry rich, and instead they should have a boring diet despite that having proved to be of no use. Opponents of THINCS counter-react that very important side effects of cholesterol lowering medications are rare. This may be interesting but possibly internet research on this subject is not very good for your own health...

A big problem in science and medical research in particular is that something that happens at the same time is being confused with causality. It is not because two things happen at the same time that one is caused by the other. If you compare enough parameters you will always find some correlations: things that happen or patterns that happen together, but are not caused by each other per se. For instance, there is a strong correlation between the use of chocolate in a country and the amount of Nobel Prize winners in that country. That is not my idea, but it was published in 2012 in the *New England Journal of Medicine* which is a very serious medical magazine. Is there something in chocolate that is making people a genius? I don't think that any sensible person will think that we can have more Western Australian Nobel Prize winners if we advise them to eat a chocolate bar every day! Or perhaps consumers in countries where the government is putting a lot of money in education and science, would they also have more money to buy chocolate? With the scientific studies to look for advantages and disadvantages of side effects of drugs there is a lot that can go wrong and as soon as a medication is allowed on the market it has to be prescribed under particular circumstances and the patient has to use it according to the advice from the doctor. On all of these fronts the problem can go wrong, and drugs can have too much effect or not enough effect or a side effect independent of the theoretic advantages. To make that clearer, here is a simple thought experiment.

Suppose it is raining heavily and a lot of people complained they had wet feet. You want to know the ins and outs of this problem, so you are going to investigate how serious it is, and what do you find? After a walk in the rain 50 out of the 100 people that walked have wet feet. You start a Facebook group "Gum Boots Against Wet Feet" and you think that will solve the problem because with gum boots people can walk in the rain without getting wet feet. So you convince half of the people that are going out for a walk to wear gum boots each time they go for a walk in the rain, and then after a while you want to check whether this initiative of yours works and what do you see? Not only 50 but now 65 people have wet feet, so you are very disappointed, and you stop the Facebook group. But then suddenly somebody comes up with the smart idea that the rain will run along the trousers into the top part of the gum boots and inside and that is why the people that wear gum boots get wet feet. Wow, why didn't I think about that myself? You are feeling better, you resurrect the Facebook group, ask them to have the gum boots on but now with little straps on the top to make sure no water can get in, and yes, they all go and walk in the rain again along with the 50 people that don't believe in the gum boots and what do we find this time? We now have 75 people that walked with wet feet. Of course, this is the end of the experiment. The gum boots are being banned and after one year everybody, 100% of the people that walk have wet feet because it is raining more severely. What nobody realises is that four of the five people that wear gum boots get sweating feet. Nobody took the trouble to analyse the type of wet feet because wet is wet right? And if you have gum boots that don't breathe in the top part you make the problem only worse because no sweat can get out. A little bit of rain that was not getting in did not make any difference. In the beginning when nobody was wearing the gum boots and it wasn't raining that hard, half of them got wet feet. From the first Facebook group 40 people wearing gum boots got sweating feet plus 25 which is half of the control group, which makes 65. Of the second Facebook group, the 50 people wearing gum boots with the top part tied off all got sweating feet, so in total now 75 people had wet feet. All this time though the gum boots were the best remedy against wet feet if the people with the gum boot would wear them only when they were going on the walk in the rain and would take out the boots when they were sitting in the restaurant having a coffee and some cakes, and if they would have put in special soles to work against sweating feet.

The wet feet are the illness, the rain is the cause. The wet road is an important risk factor. The gum boots are a working medication and sweating feet is a frequent side effect. Getting rain in the gum boots from the top part is not an important risk factor. To close the gum boots off from the top part is a change in treatment that makes the side effect only worse. Putting a special insert in the gum boot however is a simple way to get rid of the most important side effect. To walk around puddles in the road is a lifestyle choice of managing the problem with probably not needing the medication. The way to walk is a little bit longer and it would cost a bit more effort but less money—you don't have to buy the gum boots, and just staying inside when it rains is prevention. The problem for scientific investigators is that people also get wet feet when they take a bath, when they go swimming, or whether they walk on grass, that they can also slip in a pool of water, that rain also can wet other parts of the body, and that from the sky you can also have snow or hail. In other words you have to take into account a lot of factors, and before you start your trials you have to really think about what exactly it is that you want to investigate, and how you are going to separate several causes of the same problem. And you have to be careful not to be too quick to jump to conclusions. The problem for doctors is again that people can buy their gum boots too small or too big. In the first case it will make the side effect much worse and in the second case a not very important risk factor is becoming more dangerous. But it is also a problem when they are not wearing their gum boots correctly, or not at all, or don't even buy them. And so it goes on.

Whilst we are waiting the results of ongoing trials to see what the value is of statins; it is my advice that you take a statin when the doctor advises you to. But you also, together with your doctor, keep a good eye on possible side effects. As far as the risks of cholesterol are concerned, I would play safe and choose "good fats" as you find in good olive oil, avocados, and some kinds of fish. But it is clear you can also do other things to prevent heart and blood vessel disease or to counteract it if you have a problem. More activities and ceasing smoking are definitely part of that strategy.

Familial hypercholesterolaemia

Familial hypercholesterolaemia is a disease that increases your LDL levels enormously. Patients with familial hypercholesterolaemia have mutations in the LDL receptor gene which stimulates the receptors which normally take the LDL out of the blood. People with one normal and one abnormal copy of that gene have a high risk of getting heart and blood vessel problems prematurely, usually between 30 and 40 years of age. If they have two abnormal copies, then they can already have a problem when they are children and have a problem before they are 20 by having a heart attack. That is a very rare form of familial hypercholesterolaemia (one in a million babies) and that is lucky because it cannot usually be treated with cholesterol lowering medication. In those people the LDL has to be removed from the blood like a kidney dialysis, or they have to get a liver transplantation. Familial hypercholesterolaemia is a genetic problem that is sometimes not always diagnosed and is therefore often untreated. A lot of doctors think that it is a rare disease, but recent studies show that one in 250 people have familial hypercholesterolaemia, the mild form with only one abnormal copy of the gene.

7 ANGINA PECTORIS AND NARROWING OF YOUR CORONARY ARTERIES

Pain in your chest, and then suddenly whilst walking into the wind you get a very tight feeling there, as if a stone is weighing down your chest and your breathing. This usually means panic, but perhaps you have the most common heart disease in the world. They have different names. But for doctors it means that there is not enough blood going through the heart muscle which is called ischaemia and the syndrome is called angina pectoris. The pain or the feeling you have with angina pectoris is not necessarily in your throat, but you feel your chest is being compressed. The feeling is behind your breastbone, (your sternum) and often radiates not only to the bottom part of your chin but also towards your left arm. There are two different forms of angina pectoris—a stable one and an unstable one. The unstable one, the most dangerous one, sometimes looks like a heart attack or myocardial infarction. The stable one is definitely less acute, but you still need to have treatment and monitoring. Patients who know that they have stable angina pectoris need to make sure that they always have their medication at hand. Some doctors say that angina pectoris is only a symptom and not a disease and they are right, but usually we do mean that it is caused by a narrowing in the coronary artery. Just one exception of this is what we call Prinzmetal angina which is a form occurring especially in women, not because there is necessarily a significant narrowing but more because the coronary artery has spasms that causes blood obstruction, and hence the complaints.

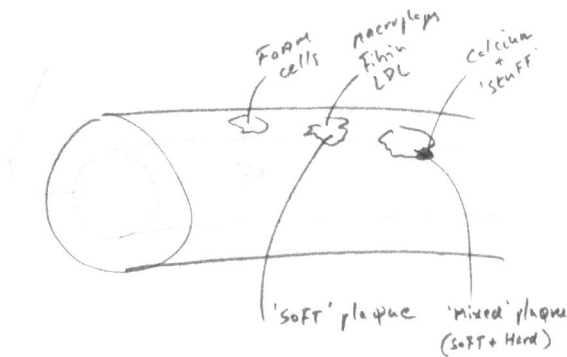

4. Schematic drawing of a coronary artery. Atherosclerotic plaque starts inside the wall of the artery with the formation of different cells, like foam cells, macrophages etc. The plaque structure is very complicated, so I often call it 'rubbish' or 'stuff'. It is important to realize that only about 15% of the plaque contains cholesterol particles. When there is no calcium deposit inside the plaque, we call it 'soft plaque'. The majority of heart attacks occur because of a problem with soft plaque. When there is calcium in the plaque (usually covering the cap of the plaque and stabilising it) we call it a calcified, hard plaque. This type of plaque is usually responsible for stable angina complaints (See text).

Diabetes and being a woman are special risk factors

The risk factors of angina pectoris are exactly the same as those for atherosclerosis in general. One of the factors is diabetes and for people with diabetes there is a little "but", because sometimes they don't feel chest discomfort when the heart does not get enough oxygen. Also women have to be careful when we consider angina pectoris because when it happens to women they do not always feel it in the chest but more generalised complaints like fatigue or dizziness or pain in the back between the shoulder blades, or being short of breath. So we know already that heart disease manifests itself differently in women compared to men and that is the reason why narrowing's in the coronary arteries in women is sometimes not recognised in time.

How do you know?

The first time that it happens it usually starts with symptoms occurring during physical exertion during work or during little jobs around the house, perhaps during sporting activities or after a big meal. In all these cases the heart is pumping and beating faster so it needs extra oxygen and that cannot be delivered because one of the channels delivering the blood (coronary arteries) are narrowed. The way people experience this feeling can differ, women not only sometimes describe their pain differently to men, but the complaints can also vary independent of gender. What one patient feels as a big rock in the middle of the chest or an elephant sitting on the chest is for another person an unpleasant feeling. Elderly patients and people with diabetes are also known to react atypically. Also the possible radiation is different, often to the lower jaw and left arm where it can also radiate to the shoulder blades, the back, the stomach, or the right arm, and sometimes it is associated with being nauseated or excessive sweating. When the heart does not need any more oxygen, then the panic or the discomfort goes away. People rest for a couple of minutes and the complaints disappear. If the complaints however, even at rest, last longer than a couple of minutes and does not disappear then they could be having a heart attack. As the narrowing's get worse and worse the pain will come faster with less exercise or even during rest. Sometimes the pain can also be more severe and last longer, and that is also the case if a narrowing in a coronary artery suddenly becomes more severe because of the occurrence of a small blood clot on that particular narrowing. If a coronary artery gets completely occluded, then we talk about a heart attack.

What angina pectoris is not?

Angina pectoris is sometimes confused with other problems. Angina is not a heart attack because there are no dying heart muscle cells, but angina pectoris can be a warning sign of a pending heart attack. Unstable angina pectoris is by the way, part of a syndrome called acute coronary syndrome because it very often results in a heart attack. There are also different diseases of the heart that can give similar sensations like certain heart valve problems or arrhythmias, but also problems with the lungs, the muscles of the chest, the stomach, or the oesophagus, can cause sudden pain in the chest like reflux or indigestion or an anxiety attack. You should always suspect a heart attack with sudden chest pain, and an extra alarm signal is if the person who is having the complaint is using their fists on the chest to explain what he is feeling. This is the so-called "sign of Levine". Levine was a famous American Cardiologist from the last century so when you have these signs and symptoms immediately present to a doctor.

8 DIAGNOSIS

The doctors usually take a picture of the electrical activity of the heart, the so-called ECG, when the patient has or has had complaints. You can't always see angina pectoris on an ECG at rest and sometimes not even when you combine it with an exercise test. If you really want to know, you might need to have a myocardial perfusion scan which you do in a nuclear medicine facility. In the hospital we can also do a cardiac catheterisation where we take films of the arteries supplying the heart with blood by putting in contrast material locally or sometimes with a CT scan where we also can get similar pictures.

How to deal with angina pectoris and live with it

The doctor can try to treat angina pectoris with nitroglycerin which is a drug that dilates blood vessels, and we can administer through a tablet or a spray under the tongue, or sometimes with a plaster on the skin. The doctor can prescribe a blood pressure lowering drug so that the heart is quieter and has less oxygen. It can also give drugs to make the blood thin which lowers the risk of an embolic process (blood clot). Most people with stable angina pectoris can have a reasonably normal life if they don't smoke, eat healthily, sleep enough, and have enough exercise.

Sports and sex

You can only do physical exercise and sport with stable angina if you discuss it with your doctor. Ideal are those activities that you can do without over-exertion like working in the garden, walking, cycling, swimming, playing golf, or aqua gym. If you suffer from unstable angina, we first need to manage the narrowing's in the arteries before you can do any exercise. The same is true for having sex. When you suffer from stable angina pectoris making love is usually no problem. You can as a prevention take nitroglycerin before you start to avoid an attack. All in all, an angina pectoris attack during sexual interaction is pretty rare in people with stable angina pectoris. You do have to note that medications like beta blocking agents can cause erectile dysfunction and that some women suffer from a dry vagina. Usually those problems are temporary. I would encourage you to discuss these issues with your doctor. I know it is not always easy but there is a good chance that they can help and that you can still have a rewarding sex life.

Driving a car

Again, with stable angina pectoris there is in principle, no objections to driving a car. If you still get an angina attack whilst driving, then pull your car along the side, put the emergency lights on, and take a nitroglycerin tablet or a spray and wait until it passes. If you have unstable angina, then you should not drive a car.

More drastic methods!

If medications or a healthy lifestyle doesn't work, then you might need something else to solve the narrowing of the arteries. That would mean doing an intervention by opening up the narrowing with a balloon, a stent, or bypass the whole troubled area in your blood vessels by doing bypass surgery.

Percutaneous transluminal coronary angioplasty

This is doctor's lingo which means the enlargement of the narrowing in a blood vessel. It happens by taking a little catheter through the skin into the blood vessel all the way up to the coronary arteries at the heart side. The term angioplasty or Dotter is named after a Mr Charles Dotter, a famous American Vascular Radiologist who invented the method in the 1960s. This procedure is not exclusively used for the heart but can be used anywhere in the body where you have a hollow organ like a blood vessel or the oesophagus or a urinary tract with a narrowing. Not everybody is a candidate for an angioplasty. The arteries can be too small or too big. Through a small opening in the groin, the doctor puts a very thin catheter through the left or right artery in the leg, a technique called cardiac catheterisation. The procedure can also be done through the inside of the elbow or through the artery in your pulse. At the end of the little tube is a small empty balloon. The doctor knows where the balloon is going by looking at the x-ray image that is being taken at the same time. Once the balloon is put at the site of the narrowing, they can inflate the balloon for a couple seconds. The plaque is being squashed into the outside of the blood vessel with the result that the diameter of the artery gets larger. At that particular moment, the blood vessel is of course completely blocked by the balloon so patients can feel some chest discomfort like their angina pectoris which is then normal. As soon as the balloon is deflated and enough blood can go through, the pain will disappear. Whether the procedure was successful is something the Cardiologist can see immediately on the monitor because he will inject a little bit of contrast material to visualise the blood flow. He can also measure the actual flow with a little Doppler catheter. If there is the notion that the artery might be recoiling and the narrowing is coming back, the doctor can decide to put in a little stent which is a little spring to keep the artery open. Usually an angioplasty takes 30 minutes to an hour but there is a lot of work to be done before and also after the treatment. Before the treatment, the doctor will explain which drugs to take and which drugs you have to (temporarily) stop. On the day of the treatment you have to be fasting. When you arrive in the hospital for your treatment, they might take some more blood tests and they might take an electrocardiogram to have the most recent details. In the room where the catheterisation is being done, the Cardiac Catheterisation Lab, you receive an infusion to protect your kidneys and for some of the medications you might need during the treatment. They will put some electrodes on your chest to measure your heart action before, during, and after the procedure, and to monitor your heartbeat. You have some local anaesthetic so that you don't feel a lot during the procedure. After the procedure, the entry point into your body is closed by putting some manual pressure on it or sometimes, we have a little gadget that will close the blood vessel. You are brought back to an observational ward where they check your heartbeat, your blood pressure, and the entry point of the procedure. They usually keep you in hospital for a couple of hours after the procedure before you are allowed to go home. You can eat but especially important is that you drink a lot so that the contrast material used during the investigation is going to be diluted and can be removed by your kidneys quicker. In most hospitals the procedure is a day procedure so you can go home the same day.

Stenting

If during the angioplasty procedure the Cardiologist is having doubts whether the inflation of the balloon will work long term, then he can also put in a very little spring at the site of the narrowing. The stent is named after Mr Charles Stent, a dentist from London, who patented a new technique in the 19th century to make tooth impressions. The function of the stent is to keep the artery open after the angioplasty balloon has been removed. It is made of metal or artificial material and is comparable with a little inverted stocking. The closed stent is put on the empty balloon and then put into the artery at the site of the narrowing, then the balloon is inflated to the right diameter with the stent on top and the stent then stays there when the balloon is deflated and removed. There are also stents made of material with a memory and they will take a predetermined diameter at the temperature of 37 degrees. The challenge with a stent is, as it is a foreign body that it doesn't cause inflammatory reactions or little blood clots because if that would happen you have a new narrowing and another problem. To reduce that risk drug eluting stents were invented. These are stents on which they have coated a small amount of drug which is slowly diffused into the tissue surrounding the stent. There are also drug coated balloons. In some countries the value of a coated stent is questioned as they are twice the price of a normal stent and the coated stent is thought to have not that much more advantages over a non-coated stent, as the post treatment with drugs is very similar for both stents. In my opinion, it is best to follow the advice of your Cardiologist because one patient is not the same as the other and that probably will determine which type of stent is the best one for that particular person in those circumstances. It depends on the bleeding risk of somebody and other possible procedures that the patient is most likely needing to have done.

9 BYPASS

Sometimes percutaneous angioplasty or stenting is not an option, for instance if the Cardiologist feels the narrowing's in the arteries are too bad or too many. That is then the reason they offer you bypass surgery, although this is more invasive. To bypass means to go around and that is exactly what is happening. The surgeon is going around the narrowing in the blood vessel because he is putting a new blood vessel alongside it. The narrowing is bridged. It is like you are in a traffic jam and you take an alternative route. In the days or weeks before the surgery they will look into more detail of the function of your heart and your coronary arteries with a blood test, an ECG, and an angiogram. You have to cease smoking and perhaps adjust your feeding patterns/lifestyle and/or your medication. The surgery itself usually takes a couple of hours depending on the technique they use. Until the end of the last century (!) the heart was always stopped for the surgery and therefore the patient had to be connected to a heart-lung machine so that the blood could continue to flow and be oxygenated. In today's world it still happens in this fashion but there are more and more bypass surgeries done on a beating heart with the use of a stabilisation system. We call this procedure an "OPCAB" which is the acronym of "off pump coronary bypass" whereby the word pump is not referring to the heart itself but the heart-lung machine. To operate on a beating heart has very important advantages: more patients survive the surgery, they have less problems with memory loss or being confused after the surgery, and they can often also shorten their stay in hospital. We see a similar evolution in scarring and the approach during the surgery. In the old days you always had to split the sternum (breast bone) for bypass surgery, nowadays they can do that with a horizontal incision between your ribcage or with a minimal invasive operation using some keyholes and a robot. There are different ways to bypass a narrowing in your coronary artery. The most important are the so-called arterial grafts (an organ or a piece of tissue that is being transplanted), a method using the left internal mammary artery (LIMA) and the one with the variant of the right side (RIMA). With the use of a venous graft (venous refers to veins), the surgeon takes a piece of vein outside the inner thigh of your leg. The length of that piece depends on the amount of narrowing's you need to bridge. That usually varies from one to five, but the record is nine! Subsequently the graft is connected on one side on the aorta or a side branch of the aorta, and the other end is put in the place of the coronary artery that is downstream from the narrowing. The transplanted vein is then used as an artery. When we use a LIMA or RIMA bypass, we take an artery from the chest wall and couple it to the diseased coronary artery, again after the narrowing that is being bypassed. In some patients it can also be done with a piece of artery from the lower arm. In any case if you use an artery as a bypass the beneficial effect of the surgery lasts longer than when you use a vein, but also with a normal vein graft, the majority of patients are still alive ten years after the surgery.

When you have to undergo coronary artery bypass grafting you are completely anaesthetised. When they do the open-heart surgery the surgeon opens your chest by using a little saw to cut through your breastbone. Potentially your heart is temporarily stopped, and you are connected to the heart-lung machine. That stopping of the heart is done by cooling the blood and by giving you an injection with a special potassium solution. After this the surgeon "harvests the graft", an artery from your chest or your arm or a vein out of your leg and then he starts the procedure of connecting it behind the narrowing or narrowing's. You will be disconnected from the heart-lung machine and your heart starts to beat by itself or perhaps it needs starting up and brought back into normal rhythm with an electrical shock or medication. The chest is closed and you get a couple of tubes in your body, usually a catheter in your bladder for your urine, an infusion in your arm or your neck to give medication, and little tubes to get rid of the fluid that was accumulated in your chest wall during the surgery. After you wake up from the anaesthetic, you feel groggy and you have to stay at least another day in the Intensive Care Unit so that the doctors can check whether your heart and your breathing are working properly. The first two or three days after the surgery you might feel that your chest is painful, but you receive medication for that. Twenty-four hours after the operation you can usually leave the Intensive Care Unit and a day later you can start walking and eating and going to the toilet yourself. Within the week you lose all your little tubes and can go home if there are no complications. To eat and sleep can be difficult for the next couple of weeks and maybe your leg is swollen and painful if they used it to harvest a vein. That is all quite normal. After a month or so you can do office work or non-strenuous activities. For heavy physical work you usually need a little bit more time. Between two to three months after the surgery you should be back to your old self.

Bypass surgeries have been done since the 1960s, by now in more than tens of millions of patients. The technique is very solid and often very successful, but there are still risks: blood clots, infections, heart rhythm problems, problems with breathing, fever, pain, lack of memory, and confusion. All these things can happen after bypass surgery depending on your age, the number of bypasses needed, the length of the operation, the technique used for the operation, and other diseases (co-morbidities) that you might have. Most of these complications can be dealt with. As we are performing more and more bypass surgeries on the beating heart and using a smaller entry point in the chest, also the rehabilitation of many more patients will be faster and with less complications. After the surgery patients are advised to follow a rehabilitation program to adjust their lifestyle and to be diligent in taking the necessary medications. If they don't then they are increasing their risk that the recuperation phase is going to be very slow and in the future that another blood vessel will narrow or narrow further or that even the bypass just made is going to be occluded prematurely.

Heart attack is always serious!

When you suffer a heart attack, a part of your heart muscle is irreversibly damaged by lack of oxygen. This area changes into a scar that cannot contribute to the pump function of the heart. The larger the scar, the smaller the chance you survive it. Also, the area where it occurs is important. If the heart attack happens in the left ventricle which is the strongest part of the heart, then that is in general much more serious than when it is in the right ventricle. But there is no such thing as a light heart attack. Even in the most favourable situation a heart attack is a very serious matter.

More than half survive it

One of the greatest misunderstandings about heart attacks is they are deadly all the time. There are no reliable accurate data on the amount of heart attacks in our country but there are annually approximately just over 15,000 people a year who have an acute myocardial infarction, usually with an average age of around 65 years. That is around

40 people a day, and more than half of those people survive the attack. The death rate by myocardial infarction in patients who arrive in hospital alive has been remarkably low in last couple of years. From a Dutch investigation with almost 15,000 patients, they found that the death rate of a large myocardial infarction in the period 2000 to 2011 is reduced to 6% as opposed to 13% ten years before that and 70% in the time between 1985 and 1990. There has been an 80% reduction in deaths in the first month after admission since 1985. Heart attack is now better recognised by people, but they are also treated faster and better. Even in the ambulance the difference between a large or a small heart attack can be made and after the initial treatment. Patients are also getting improved medications nowadays.

Symptoms

The symptoms of a heart attack are approximately the same as that of angina pectoris, both caused by underlying narrowing in your coronary arteries . You feel pressure behind your sternum (your breastbone) and an acute pain that sometimes radiates to the shoulders, usually to the left side. The pain does not come in waves but is persistent. The patient is often sweating, looks very pale, and sometimes feels nauseated. Indeed, very similar as with cases of angina pectoris, but the pain of an infarct usually lasts longer. The difference between a narrowing and an occlusion—between a lack of oxygen and no oxygen at all—can often be made with certainty only afterwards. Just like a normal attack of angina pectoris, a heart attack often has different, misleading or less severe symptoms in women, aged people, and people with diabetes. Sometimes heart attacks are silent infarcts. These ones are not recognised, often because there is only very little heart muscle involved and there are less symptoms because of that, or because people have that many other health problems like diabetes that the heart attack is not recognised or is confused with something else. Sometimes when people are investigated for other reasons years after the heart attack, they will find that a patient had one.

It often happens in the morning

In general people feel that the risk of a heart attack varies according to the timing, so there are some studies that suggest that the risk of having a heart attack is highest on a Monday morning in autumn or winter. Heart attacks are definitely more frequent before noon than compared to the rest of the day. The amount of infarcts suddenly rise between 6 and 8 o'clock in the morning, are high until approximately 11 o'clock in the morning and then slow down until 6 o'clock in the afternoon. From there, it stays very low until the early morning again. Which mechanisms are causing this we don't know exactly, but often the body requires more oxygen when it rises up but just before changing to be ready for the activities of the day, and this phenomena influence your risk of a heart attack. So having a heart attack does not necessarily depend on your specific activities on whatever day, the pattern also works on your body clock as if the heart is already getting excited even before you have done anything.

When do you need to go and see the doctor?

Every minute counts! Somebody who is suffering from a myocardial infarction but is conscious needs to be moved as quickly as possible to a doctor or a hospital. Even with the slightest hunch you must go. Even though the person might recuperate quickly. If a person is suddenly blacking out and is not reacting, then even every second counts and the sufferer needs to get CPR immediately whilst somebody else calls the emergency number.

10 IN THE HOSPITAL OR ON THE ROAD? (WHEN IT HAPPENS)

When we suspect a myocardial infarction or a heart attack, we immediately try to take an ECG. On this piece of paper you often see not only whether there is a heart attack but also where the heart attack is located, for instance in the front part of heart or the back part of the heart, or maybe bottom part of the heart. If the doctor sees that the line between the point S and point T of the ECG is elevated it is called a STEMI, which is the abbreviation of ST elevation myocardial infarction. In all other cases we deal with a non-STEMI. This is an important difference because a lot of patients with a STEMI are currently brought into the cardiac catheterization suite straight away where a percutaneous transluminal coronary angioplasty (PTCA or balloon procedure) can be performed to open up the narrow blood vessel. While if you suffer from a non-STEMI, they first want to perform an echocardiogram of the heart or a nuclear study to be better informed about what the best treatment for the patient would be. Time is money. The faster a closure of the coronary arteries is being resolved the smaller is the damage to the 'engine'. If the closure is relieved within two hours of its occurrence, then the extent of damage could be reduced more than 50%. If you are able to do it within six hours you can save up to one third of the jeopardized heart muscle. In the "older days", the treatment of a heart attack occurred with thrombolysis which is the administration of a medicine which can resolve blood clots. In the meantime, we know that opening up the blood vessel with a balloon is better and safer, but this depends whether the patient arrives at the hospital on time—usually within one and a half hours of the onset of complaints—where a PTCA can be performed. In Western Australia in the city of Perth and immediate suburbs that is possible, however anything outside the one-and-a-half-hour time frame like in cities such as Geraldton, Kalgoorlie, Broome, Esperance, we have to use the thrombolysis. For very severe narrowing's or a chain of narrowing's, often a bypass surgical procedure is necessary. No matter how you look at it, the treatment of a heart attack has dramatically changed in the last 10 to 20 years. In the old days, you had to rest a lot and get strong again which would usually take longer than a month. Really, you only got worse from that, and in the meantime the patient took medication to thin the blood to try to prevent the next attack. In today's world, the coronary artery is opened up as quickly as possible and you are encouraged to act as normal as possible as quickly as possible. Hospitals often have their own cardiac rehabilitation unit to facilitate that and you still need lots of medication to counter any new blood clots, against cholesterol levels, and against high blood pressure.

Causes

A heart attack is mostly caused by a new blood clot on top of an atheroma in a coronary artery. That causes a blood clot which blocks the blood flow, or the blood clot breaks off and lodges more downstream, and then it means that a previously not significant narrowing suddenly evolves into a complete occlusion. Infarct is from the Latin language from the verb "infarcire" which means to occlude. Atheromatous plaques have two ways to lead to an infarct—number one is that it can rupture and therefore cause a blood clot, and the second option is that they grow so much that they actually cause a narrowing of the coronary artery to such a degree that even a very small blood clot can cause a complete occlusion. Atherosclerosis is the main culprit. We have already discussed the risk factors for atherosclerosis : age, smoking and passive smoking, high blood pressure, too many kilos, too much LDL cholesterol and triglycerides, diabetes, familial history (genetics), and a lack of exercise. A much rarer form of a heart attack without even atherosclerosis can occur and is called the spontaneous dissection of a coronary artery. In this case there is a rupture in the inner lining of the artery, the so-called tunica intima. We don't know exactly what causes the little tear. Perhaps it has to do with an abnormality in the connective tissue built up in that person. Of note is that this problem predominantly occurs in females, often after giving birth or around the menopause. This suggests that perhaps there are hormonal factors in play here as well. Another possible cause would be that a little blood clot from the left ventricle is "getting lost" in the coronary artery.

The coronary artery is the first side branch of the aorta when the blood leaves the heart. This can sometimes occur in patients with atrial fibrillation. That abnormality of the rhythm is now acutely dangerous because only the top part of the heart, the atria, are contracting randomly and the ventricles are doing their work normally. However, because of the irregular contractions the normal blood flow which is in essence a parallel going stream like the middle of a fast flowing river, is disturbed and the small turbulences that occur pose a risk for the occurrence of small blood clots. Such a little blood clot can travel from the left ventricle and the aorta in the coronary artery, and in the worst-case scenario occlude it straight away. The fourth option is that vasculitis or an inflammation of the artery can cause a heart attack. One form of vasculitis is the disease of Kawasaki, not the motor cycle but an infection in children which can cause a coronary artery to inflame to such a degree that it bursts, so even kids can have a heart attack although that is extremely rare!

Consequences and complications

In the best scenario the patient will be able to receive medical assistance quickly and only a small part of the heart will be damaged, but even then a heart attack is a physical and spiritual event that can really change the life of the patient and the patient's environment. All kinds of tests are being done, a lot of pills have to be taken, important lifestyle changes are in order, and sometimes operations have to take place. Yes, you are looking death in the eyes even when you just hear the word heart attack. You have of course people that are very stoic and are very quickly back into their old habits after they suffered a heart attack, but for most people who survive a heart attack it is a real wake up call. In the worse cases of heart attack, life threatening complications can occur, immediately, during, and after the heart attack, but also at a later stage.

Ventricular fibrillation and cardiac stand still

If people die from a heart attack, the cause is often ventricular fibrillation. People who watch American television series will know that this event is known as ventricular fib. As soon as you hear that cry on the ER, everything goes into mayhem. Ventricular fibrillation is a life-threatening situation where the heart chambers are not contracting any more. The heart is still moving but is no longer contracting. The pump function is gone. There is no blood flow, the tissues like the heart itself, but also the brain and the lungs are not getting oxygen. Within ten seconds you are unconscious, within five minutes you have irreversible brain damage, and after ten minutes you are biologically dead. You can only solve ventricular fibrillation by defibrillating the heart. You do this with a defibrillator in the hospital or with an automatic external defibrillator (AED) as you find often but still not often enough in public spaces. In any case, whilst you are waiting for a defibrillator only cardiac massage can keep the life of that person going until the ambulance has arrived. We will discuss cardiac massage and CPR in the last chapter, but the essence is that only five to ten percent of people that suffer ventricular fibrillation outside the hospital survive the episode, and that is often because when it occurs there is nobody around, but if somebody is around we need to know what we should do and the guts to do it. If somebody suddenly falls to the ground, is not reacting to any stimuli, and is not breathing normally, then potentially you talk about a ventricular fibrillation and acute loss of life is imminent. You don't have to know much to give that life another chance. You can call ooo or have somebody call it, you can yourself restart the heart by connecting a defibrillator, or you can start heart massage by pushing on the middle of the chest rhythmically approximately 5cm in and then out in the beat of the song "Staying Alive" by the Bee Gees. By the way, the automatic external defibrillators which you find in public places are completely automatic. In the Netherlands and Belgium, they developed a drone defibrillator that will be at the scene much quicker than the ambulance who has to use the road. It is completely automated as you can get instructions from the operator on the other side of the camera.

Heart failure

If a myocardial infarction has damaged the large part of the heart muscle, then the patient can die acutely or can get chronic heart failure. In the case of heart failure, the pump is still working but not good enough to get the required blood into the tissues.

Heart valve problems

A heart attack can cause the mitral valve between the left ventricle and the left atrium to leak. This valve is connected with little tendons at the site of the left ventricle, and especially when the back part of the heart has suffered an infarct the back leaflet of the mitral valve is sometimes just hanging there because the tendons don't work. This causes the mitral valve not to close properly. If part of the heart that supplies the tendons with oxygen has died then these tendons can rupture a couple of days after the heart attack as well, and then suddenly a large mitral insufficiency is caused which also can enhance the chances of sudden death.

Rupture

The left ventricular wall can also rupture itself. If that happens the patient almost always dies. If there is a rupture between the left and the right side, the survival rate is a little bit better, but still 70 to 80% of people in which this happens will die. A little tear in the heart muscle can cause the pericardial sac around the heart to fill up with blood which prohibits the heart from pumping properly as well. This is called tamponade.

Cardiac tamponade

If there is a cardiac tamponade the heart cannot get enough blood into the right side of the heart during the rest phase of the heart cycle and that is because there is fluid around the heart in the pericardial sac. This fluid presses on the heart and prohibits the heart to relax and fill with blood again. The patient will get short of breath and turn blue. In severe cases it can cause death. Heart tamponade can be caused by a trauma, cancer, kidney failure, inflammation of the pericardial sac, but also as complication of an operation, a rupture of the cardiac muscle often in the first couple of days after the occurrence of a heart attack.

11 WARNING LIGHTS?

A lot has been written about the question whether you can feel a heart attack or a myocardial infarction coming. Well let me be very clear on this: most heart attacks happen as thunder in a clear sky... But if you listen carefully to people who went through the experience and you ask the right questions, you will find that in the period of approximately four weeks until maybe only one hour before the occurrence of the myocardial infarction, there are smaller or sometimes larger signs that predicted it, and you will find that for whatever reason those people did not pay the appropriate attention to the signals. The truth is that most heart attacks start slowly with mild discomfort or pain. That is in itself not illogical. A heart attack is just a late phase of the slow progression of atherosclerosis. Your damaged coronary arteries are closing up just a little bit further every day and every night if you don't do anything about it. That means the blood can get less and less easily through the narrowing and then suddenly on one given time and moment there no more blood is going through there, but that can occur weeks, days or only hours after the moment that just a little bit of blood is going through. That particular moment was on the horizon and your heart did try to acknowledge it and to try to warn you that you had a problem. It's as if your engine suddenly sputters and refuses to work anymore when you are low on petrol being a surprise, if you don't pay attention to your fuel gauge this will happen to your heart as well.

Think about warning signs like unexplained tiredness, something you hear very often, or an unpleasant pressing feeling on your chest, pain in your arms, your back, your neck, your jaw, perhaps your stomach, being short of breath without doing any exercise, or a prolonged period of shortness of breath after exercise is also questionable, whether that is in combination with chest discomfort or chest pain or not. Other possible warning signs are cold sweat, palpitations, nausea, dizziness, and a very persistent hiccough. Sure, these are relatively vague signals and everybody sometimes has a funny feeling but you still have to look at the dashboard of your body and see whether your fuel gauge is in the right place, and if you can't find a good reason for your complaints, then it is better to have a chat to your GP or go to the Emergency Department of your hospital, or call an ambulance. Better safe than sorry. If in the end they find that everything is OK, then that will be very good news and good luck.

What do I do when I am alone?

If you think or fear that you are having or going to have a heart attack and you are by yourself then call an ambulance and move as little as possible so you are not putting extra stress on your heart. If it happens when you are on the road, first go and park on the side of the road. Don't try to drive to a hospital yourself. You can become unconscious and you can kill yourself or others. If you are already on a beta blocking agent (medication that you usually have for treatment of high blood pressure) and you have it handy then take a tablet.

Is it your first attack? Then take an Aspirin as quickly as possible. Put it in your mouth, chew on it and swallow it. Aspirin is a good drug against little blood clots. Scientists found a long time ago what would work the fastest. An Aspirin taken with some water or chewed for 30 seconds and then drink it. It was a small experiment but chewing it gave the fastest result. You can also use these tips if somebody in your neighbourhood thinks they are having a heart attack. If that person does not lose consciousness, if they do not react to stimuli, or they are barely breathing, then possibly it is already a stopping of the heart due to ventricular fibrillation and you have to start your CPR straight away. To deliver Aspirin or other medication is something you don't have to think about at that moment. Maybe you are now thinking about taking an Aspirin preventative every day to prevent a heart attack just in case. In Australia you can buy low dose Aspirin over the counter, but I think it is still better to discuss this with your GP or your Cardiologist before you decide to do that. Aspirin is a drug and it is not there for everybody. It can have side effects and don't forget, the fact that you can buy it over the counter doesn't mean that it is safe for everybody, it has risks.

Pain in the leg syndrome and peripheral vascular disease

Another possible cause of consequence of arterial disease, less dramatic than a heart attack but still very frequent, is the phenomena of painful legs. The painful legs were described first by a German author and it was called "Schaufenster krankheit". A Schaufenster is a German word for a shop window and what happened was that people with pain in their legs would walk down the street, get a terrible pain in the leg, and had to stand still to wait for it to subside, so they turned to the window of a shop pretending to study the content while they were waiting for the pain to subside. It is also called smokers' legs because it is a very frequent disease occurring in people that smoke. Together with diabetes, smoking is the most important cause of this problem. This type of peripheral vascular disease problem is found five times more often in people that smoke than people who do not smoke. It is more prevalent in men as compared to women. These complaints are the most known symptom of peripheral vascular disease which is a disease that does not give any symptoms in two thirds of all patients that have it. Peripheral means far away from the heart and more specifically in the legs. There are different statistics about this but probably in the age group between 50 to 60 years of age you would see 5% of the population having peripheral arterial disease. If you are over 80 it is more than 25%. In medicine and in medical books you will find a phenomena known as "claudicatio intermittens" which means being a cripple at intervals, and it is called that because patients with atherosclerosis of one of the arteries to the legs or in both legs get pain when they walk, and they have to pause and stand still every couple of minutes, just like when people are shopping. Usually they complain about pain in the calf muscle and the reason for that is the same as with angina pectoris: lack of oxygen in the muscle. During walking, and we are not talking about running but just walking, the leg muscles need more oxygen, but because they do not get enough blood, there is more production of lactic acid, and the lactic acid causes a cramp that will go away when you stop and there is a little bit of improvement to the blood supply.

What you can you do yourself?

If when you walk you get a pain in your leg once in a while which improves quickly when you rest, then you can possibly deal with the problem yourself by changing your lifestyle. Maybe you could eat less bad fatty food, maybe you could exercise more, and if you smoke, you stop. Stopping smoking probably has more effect than all medications taken together.

When do you have to see a doctor?

You can measure the seriousness and the development of your problem yourself by looking at the distance that you can walk without pain. If you still have complaints or they are getting worse, the best thing you can do is consult your doctor. It is important that you seek help with this condition because without any treatment you will eventually get pain when you are not walking and sitting in a chair. The end game is that you do not get enough oxygen in your muscles at all and you get gangrene. If you tackle peripheral vascular disease early enough an operation is seldom necessary, and if you do that not only the arteries going to your legs, but all your arteries including your coronary arteries will feel better. Peripheral vascular disease often coincides with heart and other blood vessel problems which at that time might not be obvious. In this sense the occurrence of symptomatic peripheral vascular disease could be an early warning sign and dealing with it can not only save your leg but probably your life.

How can medical science help?

The doctor can diagnose your peripheral vascular disease. It can be confusing because some people with ischias, a nerve problem that starts in the back, can be difficult to differentiate. The doctor can measure an arm-ankle index, sometimes they will do an angiogram, a physiotherapist can help you with a walking or jogging program which can help to reduce your complaints or even make them go away. Sometimes you get advice to take medicine for the pain but also to improve the blood supply as an adjunctive to a healthier lifestyle. There is no medicine that can work like a magic bullet to make the atherosclerosis disappear. Surgery should be your last resort but if the other options do not do the job, a specialist can try to deal with the narrowing by dilatation with a balloon and/or in combination with a stent. In some cases, they can make a bypass with a piece of artery that taken from somewhere else in your body or with an artificial artery.

Aorto-bi-femoral bypass

An aorto-bi-femoral bypass is a surgical procedure to create a new path around the large clogged blood vessels in your abdomen or groin. This procedure involves placing a graft to bypass the clogged blood vessel. The graft is an artificial conduit. One end of the graft is surgically connected to your aorta before the blocked or diseased section, the other ends of the graft are each attached to one of your femoral arteries after the blocked or diseased section. This graft redirects the blood flow and allows the blood to continue flowing past the blockage. We can offer this technique if ballooning or stenting does not help any more. There are several types of bypass procedures and the aorta or bi-femoral bypass is specifically for the blood vessels that run between your aorta and the femoral arteries. In classical times, the surgeon had to cut open your whole abdomen from your chest to your pubic bone, but nowadays it also happens more and more through minimally invasive surgery where a kind of complete prosthesis is inserted.

Venous thrombosis legs and economy class!

Peripheral vascular disease is often confused with the occurrence of a deep vein thrombosis leg. In the case of a deep vein thrombosis, we have a blood clot, a so-called thrombus. The blood has a coagulation system to help us to deal with internal or external bleedings, but it is never intended that the blood within the veins or arteries is clogging. This clogging process is called thrombosis. This thrombosis is a problem if it occurs in arteries or veins. A thrombosis in an artery can be life threatening and we have discussed that already when we talked about heart attacks. But venous thrombosis also occurs and one of the most commonly known causes is a thrombosis in the legs, and sometimes in the arm. The possible symptoms of the occurrence of a thrombosis in a leg are pain, hence the probable confusion with peripheral vascular disease, but also lack of feeling like a sleeping leg, swelling, or redness. The biggest risk from a thrombosis in the leg (DVT, deep vein thrombosis) is that it will dislodge and go through the blood vessel system, through the right side of the heart into the lung, then we talk about a pulmonary embolus. The symptoms of a pulmonary embolus are usually a superficial and painful breathing pattern, and shortness of breath. DVT and pulmonary emboli often occur together and together they are a dangerous disease. A DVT can be caused by lack of movement, for instance in people who have to stay in bed for a long time because of a chronic disease, or in travellers who take long journeys in a train, car, or plane. As it was described in planes quite a few times, DVT has got the nickname of "economy class disease". The list of other risk factors is pretty long. You can have problems with your coagulation factors, especially in younger DVT patients, age, obesity, some medications like hormone therapies and/or anticonception, pregnancy, malignancy, varicose veins, operations, and severe infections. We should also not forget the effect of very sugary nutritional items. Since we have consumed more sugars and carbohydrates, the amount of DVT's has significantly increased. The diagnosis of DVT is made by means of ultrasound. The treatment consists of medication to make the blood thin with injections of Heparin, Clexane, or with tablets that have to be taken for months on end. Sometimes people are advised to have certain support stockings and exercise more. To move more does not increase your risk for a pulmonary embolism. Don't forget, the treatment of DVT is often difficult and takes a long time.

Rupture of the aorta (aortic dissection)

If somebody suddenly falls to the ground, loses consciousness, and nothing that we do works, even if some witness immediately starts CPR, then often we are dealing with a rupture of the biggest artery, the aorta. Of course, it could be a very large heart attack or an arrhythmia of the heart, but the rupture of the aorta where blood is streaming through the rupture under high pressure in the chest or the abdomen is more common. It is almost always lethal, even when it happens in hospital.

Traumatic or spontaneously?

There are two forms of an aortic rupture. One is traumatic which is usually an external trauma like a traffic accident, which is happening more often than they thought in the past. It is known that in at least 18% of fatalities in traffic accidents, the direct cause of death is a rupture of the aorta. Often it is not immediately recognized because the victim has a lot of other external wounds. A traumatic aortic rupture can also occur when people fall. This can be compared with a little balloon that you throw from the second story of the house it usually stays intact, but if you fill it with water and you throw it outside it will explode with great pressure. The usual place where the aorta ruptures is just in the top part where it bends down inside the chest, just at the area where most of the side branches occur.

With a spontaneous aortic rupture, we can identify a rupture which is not caused by an accident but usually caused by an aneurysm—a little weak spot in the wall of the aorta that over the years causes a little balloon and weak spot. It will grow over the years and then on one bad day it will burst and rupture. The few people that survive this talk about a sudden unbearable pain in the tummy or in the chest. In the latter, it is very difficult to differentiate between a large heart attack and a rupture of the aorta by the complaints alone. Bystanders will often see how the victim is suddenly very pale, collapses, and almost immediately loses consciousness. In hospital the cardiovascular surgeon can localize the rupture or the hole in the aorta and try to fix it with a prosthesis. Sometimes there is only a small hole or a partial tear. When that is the case the prognosis is indeed much better. A spontaneous aorta aneurysm can be caused because of an inflammation or from an imbalance between the proteins that make the blood vessel wall and the proteins that break down the blood vessel wall. It is more prevalent in elderly males and especially in people that smoke. Sometimes there is also a genetic factor in play like the syndrome of Marfan.

Marfan syndrome

The syndrome of Marfan, named after the French paediatrician Antoine Marfan, is a genetic disease of the collagen which is a type of tissue that occurs in many places in the body. In Marfan's it is related predominantly to the eyes, the skeleton, the heart, and the blood vessels. The incidence of the disease is two to three people out of ten thousand. Often you can see that people have Marfan because they are very tall, lean, they have their chest bone pressed inside or outside, and their fingers are that flexible that the thumb can overlap the pinkie if they have one hand over the wrist of the other. It is a typical sign. Less obvious are the eye abnormality and heart valve abnormalities. The symptoms are not always present in all Marfan patients and they can also occur one by one in people that do not have Marfan. The ultimate test is a genetic investigation. Many historical or current celebrities that have these particular features have a lot of people speculating about whether they do have Marfan, for instance Pharaoh Tutankhamun, Julius Caesar, the violin maestro Niccolo Paganini, American President Abraham Lincoln, the pianist Sergei Rachmaninoff, Osama Bin Laden, the Olympic swimmer Michael Phelps, are all possible Marfan patients. Michael Phelps has by the way, always denied it but it is a fact that long fingers and a long wingspan have definite advantages for certain musicians, athletes, or criminals. It is also a fact that people with Marfan have a higher risk to have an aortic aneurysm at a young age. That is the reason we keep them on regular follow up regimes. People with Marfan can live a very normal life. Genetics also play a role in the aorta outside the Marfan syndrome. Aortic aneurysms are more prevalent in some families, even without Marfan. Approximately 25% of people with an aortic aneurysm have one or more first degree relatives with a similar problem.

Triple AAA

Most of the aortic aneurysms are present in the abdomen, your tummy. That is the explanation for the term AAA, or abdominal aortic aneurysm. Four to eight percent of men between 65 and 80 have an AAA, in women it is four times less. All in all, an aortic aneurysm does not rupture that often, maybe 30 cases per million people. In comparison to the occurrence of heart attacks that is very low, but while in heart attack cases more than 50% survive, an AAA rupture is between 75 to 90% deadly. If the aorta ruptures while located in the chest, then the survival chance is almost zero. Maybe we should put another A in front of the AAA syndrome, the A of anonymous. Indeed, most people who survive a rupture of an AAA did not know that they had it. Even more than narrowing of the arteries an aortic aneurysm is a time bomb, but then one that doesn't tick. If an aneurysm is diagnosed early, then almost always it is by coincidence because of an investigation or surgery of another disease or trauma. The child of an acquaintance of mine which always looked like a very healthy little man had to go to hospital after a fall. It was at the Emergency Department that the doctors detected a very large aneurysm in the tummy of the boy . It was not rupturing but the surgeon said it could have at any moment. His parents didn't know anything, the boy didn't know anything, so the fall was a blessing in disguise. He has been operated on and is doing just fine.

When do you go to the doctor then, and how can a doctor help?

In rare cases an AAA gives a knocking feeling in the area of your belly button. Also pain in the back has been reported, especially when the aneurysm presses against the spine, but usually the patient doesn't feel anything. As far as prevention goes, there is not much more you can do than keeping your blood pressure in check, don't smoke, or go to your doctor if you are part of a risk group (if family members have it for instance). That is also the case if you are a man over 60 that has a high blood pressure or smoked. As our population is getting older, we will have more AAA and more ruptures. We see that already—in 2009 worldwide, approximately 100,000 people died from an AAA, in 2013 it was already 150,000. I think it would be a very good idea if all males who smoke and are older than 50 years of age would be investigated for an AAA at least once. In Britain they already do that. You do this investigation by doing an ultrasound of the aorta in the tummy. It is a quick procedure, it is very accurate, and it does not hurt. If this investigation finds a small aneurysm, the patient needs to control his blood pressure and have a check-up every two years. If the aneurysm has a diameter of 5.5cm or more (5cm for women) then the risks of an operation are lower than the risk that the aneurysm will rupture, hence a surgical procedure is planned. In that case there are two options; the aneurysm is surgically removed and you have a prosthesis which means you are in hospital between one and two weeks, or the surgeon puts a prosthesis through the blood vessel and seals off the aneurysm from the rest of the aorta, a so-called endoprosthesis. If they are able to do that you can usually go home the next day.

12 HEART VALVE PROBLEMS

What is that?

Every year some couple of thousand Australians receive the bad news that they have a problem with their heart valves. Just as a reminder, we have four heart valves: two between the top part of the heart, the atria, and the bottom part of the heart, the ventricles. We have the tricuspid valve on the right side and the mitral valve on the left side. And we also have two between the ventricles and the arteries, the pulmonic artery on the right side and the aortic valve on the left side. The mitral valve consists of two leaflets or slips, the other valves have all three leaflets. When the atria are contracting, the valves towards the ventricles have to open completely and as the ventricles are contracting then first these valves have to be completely closed and have the valves to the arteries open, and subsequently close again. It looks a little bit like the diaphragm of a photo camera. The valves themselves have no muscles. They open and close by the pressure differences in the blood stream and because of the contraction pattern of the heart. If one or more valves are not working properly then the heart tries to compensate by working extra hard to get your blood into your tissues. Abnormalities in your valve therefore cause a higher stress on the heart. Normal heart valves have to open perfectly as well as close perfectly so that there is no leakage. We can therefore differentiate two main valve problems, one is that the opening of the valves is narrowed because of calcification or adhesion of the valve leaflets, but they can also leak because of damaged, floppy, or elongated valve leaflets. In the first case there is not enough blood into the ventricles or the arteries, and the second case the blood can flow in the wrong direction. In each case the heart has to do double time.

The most important abnormalities

The most abnormalities we see in the left side of the heart are related to the mitral valve and the aortic valve. When we see aortic stenosis, the opening between the left ventricle and the aorta is too small. That can be congenital, you are born with it, or it can occur later because of rheumatism or when people get older because of calcifications of the valve. If the problem is not recognized and continues on, then it will lead to left ventricular hypertrophy which is a thickening of the wall of the muscle wall of the left ventricle.

The mitral valve can leak. In that case we talk about mitral valve incompetence or insufficiency. It can also be narrowed, and this is called mitral valve stenosis. A combination of the two is also possible. When we have mitral incompetence, the blood goes backwards from the left ventricle to the left atrium and it will even go back into the veins in the lung. That is the reason people get short of breath very fast, sometimes even at rest, and that is when we talk about congestive heart failure.

Causes

Heart valve problems can be congenital. You could have this from birth. Some babies are born with fusion of the valve leaflets or with valves which are too big or too small. That is not always obvious when the baby is born. In some cases, the problem occurs much later in life. Valve abnormalities can also occur during one's life. Just like your arteries, your valves can get calcified over the years, less flexible, and sometimes shrink a bit. But you can also have valve problems when you are younger, sometimes bacteria from other parts of the body use the bloodstream to get to the heart and damage your valve. The cause can also be in the heart itself. If your heart muscle is enlarged or dilated because of an illness, then the leaflets of the mitral and the tricuspid valve are being pulled outwards and then they cannot close anymore. The valve could also be damaged when you suffer a heart attack.

And when do you need to see a doctor?

Some valve abnormalities do not give any complaints, others do. You have to think about being tired without any exercise, shortness of breath, swollen feet, chest discomfort or dizziness when you exert yourself. If you find that you suffer from one of these symptoms you better have a chat to your GP.

How can medical science help you here?

It is possible that your GP thinks that you might have a valvular problem because he listens to your heart with his stethoscope and observes an abnormality, a murmur. You are then referred to a Cardiologist or a hospital for further investigations like an ECG, an ultrasound of heart, an MRI scan of the heart, or a cardiac catheterization. When a valvular abnormality has been diagnosed, the severity of the abnormality will dictate the advice for further treatment. Some smaller abnormalities do not need any particular treatment and are kept under surveillance regularly. Other problems can be treated with medication that lowers blood pressure or blood thinning medication. These treatments do not fix your valve but will help counteract possible deterioration of the valve problem. They have to make sure that the heart is not stressed too much. When it is found that the valve problem is serious then you must have surgery. Possibly a big surgery is needed where they have to cut open your chest and stop the heart, but other times it can be through minimally invasive surgery with a little hole between your ribs and/or through a catheter through your groin, similar to how we treat problems with coronary arteries.

To repair or exchange—that is the question

Sometimes the surgeon is able to repair a valve because he can detach valve leaflets that were fused together or he can cut away abnormal parts and fix the valve by making it smaller with a clip which is a small plastic ring. In other cases, a completely new valve is necessary. In case of an open-heart surgical procedure for a new valve, they stop the heart, then the surgeon opens the heart to get access to the valve that he is going to replace. If you are talking about changing the aortic valve, he will open the aorta, cut away the defective valve and replace it with a new one. That is an artificial valve that has usually a ring of metal and cloth which has the purpose of holding the little stitches to secure the valve in the right spot. If that has been done, the surgeon gets the blood through the coronary arteries, the heart starts to beat, and they disconnect the heart/lung machine. An artificial valve made of plastic or metal is something that you have for the rest of your life, even though they will open and close one hundred thousand times a day. The disadvantage of artificial valves is that they make ticking noises, and they destroy little blood platelets which is why you need anticoagulation for the rest of your life. This is a nuisance and it also increases your risk of a bleed. The alternative is biological valves. These are made of animal material, usually from pigs or cows, or they can come from a human donor. Biological valves make no sound and they only need the first one to three months anticoagulation, but they have another big drawback—they usually only last 15 years. Which valve to use is a choice made between patient, cardiologist, and cardiac surgeon.

Dutch scientists are currently looking for the ideal new heart valve. They already experimented with valves that were made in the laboratory by breeding a patient's own cells on a structure, but that technique would take too long and was too expensive. Currently there is another line of investigation. It might be possible in the future that we are able to introduce an artificial valve made of a porous biological material that will disintegrate itself. These are polymers a thousandth of a millimetre thin and they carry stuff that attracts a certain type of white blood cell. These cells connect themselves in and on the temporary valve. After some time on top of this, you form collagen which gives you a pretty steady structure. The implanted valve itself disintegrates and what is left in the body is a new valve made entirely with material of the body itself. This is the future, but current tests in sheep are looking very successful. Of all laboratory animals, sheep wear out their valves the fastest, so if the new valve will be successful in sheep then it might work everywhere.

And then the risks

Heart valve operations are usually very successful but as is the case with all surgeries, there are always the complication risks. For instance, if we change the aortic valve, we can damage the bundle of His and the patient needs a pacemaker. You can have a bleed in your pericardial sac, but that is usually something that the surgeon can deal with. Patients with a new heart valve have a high chance of endocarditis, a bacterial infection. That is why a lot of patients get preventative antibiotics when they have a procedure or suffer a trauma, go to the dentist for treatment or cleaning of the teeth. It is rare but it does happen that people die when they have had a new heart valve surgery, and that is the reason why doctors always discuss the pros and cons of the procedure. In case of very bad valve disease in people with a bad general condition or special risk factors, that can be a pretty difficult choice, especially because often the decision not to operate also means that the patient's life expectancy is greatly reduced.

Infections and inflammation

Myocarditis, endocarditis, pericarditis—all diseases that end with "itis" are inflammations. They are usually caused by an infection but that is not always all that is needed. There is confusion between the difference of infection and inflammation so I will explain it in short. An inflammation is a reaction of the body on damaged tissue or external influences. That could be because of micro-organisms like bacteria or viruses or parasites or fungi, but also insect bites, irritant chemical material (like medication) or radiation (heat, ironizing radiation, UV radiation etc.). Tissues can also be damaged because of an autoimmune reaction where our own immune system is wrong and thinks that some tissues are the enemy, so you can get a tendon inflammation as cause of a repetitive strain injury which is caused by making a repetitive movement for a long time. Just ask people that play computer games all the time or cashiers who work at the supermarket, or our secretaries who type letters all day. The inflammatory process can be very painful and annoying, but it has a proper goal—it wants to get rid of the offending stimulus and repair the damage done.

An infection happens when a micro-organism or another sick making bug gets into your body and has replicated itself there with or without doing damage. In other words, not all infections cause inflammation, and not all inflammatory processes are caused by an infection, and that is also true for the heart.

Myocarditis

Myocarditis is an inflammation of the heart muscle, usually caused by a virus. Other causes could be bacteria, a parasite or being sensitive to some medication, radiation or an autoimmune disease. The first symptoms are flu-like like fever and muscle pain which usually disappear. But in serious cases the disease comes back so badly that after a few weeks you have already congestive heart failure and/or serious rhythm abnormalities. Usually the myocarditis is pretty benign, and the complaints are sometimes much later which are usually confined to chronic shortness of breath and tiredness. So no myocarditis is the same, it can go either way. The treatment depends on the cause and the symptoms. Viruses are very difficult to deal with but luckily, they usually heal by themselves.

Bacterial Endocarditis

In the case of bacterial endocarditis, we have bacteria in the bloodstream, and they attack the heart and the inside of the heart, the so-called endocard, as well as the heart valves. There is also a non-infectious form of endocarditis but that one is very rare. Bacterial endocarditis is rare but very dangerous. Again, it starts with difficult to pinpoint complaints, usually flu like symptoms, and the diagnosis can sometimes be very much delayed and usually calls for more investigations. The bacteria get into the body and the blood through a little nick in the skin, the mouth, or the gums of your teeth. In normal cases our immune system can deal with the invasion, but if the immune system is not one hundred percent they can still get where we don't want them. We have a chronic form or endocarditis as well as an acute endocarditis. As soon as we make the diagnosis of bacterial endocarditis you have to get an infusion with antibiotics. The treatment usually happens in hospital and can take over a month. That treatment process usually kills off the bacteria and gets rid of the infection, but often there is damage done on the heart and the heart valves like a leaking valve, and that means that you might need to have surgery. If you don't want to get endocarditis it is important to have very good mouth hygiene and don't use intravenous drugs!

Pericarditis

Pericarditis is an inflammation of the pericardium, the little sac around the heart, and can be acute or chronic. The most usual cause of pericarditis is a virus infection after the flu or a cold, but you can also get pericarditis when you are undergoing open heart surgery or when you have a heart attack or another disease. The symptoms are very similar to those of the other inflammatory processes of the heart, first fatigue and some flu like symptoms, then chest pain, shortness of breath, and extreme tiredness. But in the case of acute pericarditis, the pain in the chest can be very severe because of the pericardium tissues rubbing against the heart. Usually the pain is more severe when you move or when you breathe in deeply or when you lie on your back. With our stethoscope we can often hear the friction of the tissues. It is a bit like two pieces of leather that you rub together. The treatment depends on the cause and the symptoms. Often it heals by itself. A special but rare form is constrictive pericarditis where the pericardium hardens after the infection and therefore is no longer flexible and cannot allow the heart to get bigger and smaller when it pumps the blood around. In those cases, the pericardium sometimes needs to be surgically removed to allow the heart muscle more space.

13 CARDIAC ARRHYTHMIAS

Cardiac arrhythmias speak for themselves. You may have this problem in many ways. Firstly, a rhythm which is faster than normal. We should really call it a tempo because tempo reflects speed and rhythm reflects regularity, and a faster rhythm than normal we call tachycardia. A rhythm which is too slow we call bradycardia. A cardiac rhythm can also be irregular, even sometimes completely chaotic, and this can happen continuously or in attacks. The seriousness also changes, it can be very innocent, it can be concerning, or it can be life-threatening or deadly.

Normal abnormal rhythms

A normal heart in rest is beating approximately 70 times per minute. If that is truly the norm then there are a lot of abnormal rhythms, however there is nothing wrong with these. Somebody's heartbeat can have a lot of normal speeds depending on the circumstances. Your heartbeat goes down if you are sleeping and goes up when you exercise. We call that exercise related tachycardia. A healthy heart can pump up to seven times more blood during a heavy exercise than compared to rest. The maximum heartbeat at exercise depends on your age. As a rule of thumb your maximal heartbeat is 220 beats per minute minus your age, so for a 40-year-old that is 180 beats per minute, but this can change per person. If you take for instance beta blocking agents, your maximum heartbeat is a lot lower. Not only during sports or heavy manual work does your heart frequency increase, but it also happens when you are frightened or when there is stress involved. The body produces extra adrenaline and nor adrenaline in those cases and that causes the heart to go a little faster as well. If your heart starts to race when you have to give a public speaking address or during a thriller on the television or on top of a ladder which is not stable, then having an increased heartbeat in those circumstances is very normal. There are lots of differences between different people, depending among others on your age and level of fitness. The average at rest of a newborn baby is not 70 but 130 beats per minute, and the heartbeat of kids going to primary school between 80 and 120, trained athletes and especially athletes doing long hauls of exercise like cyclists or marathon runners, they have usually an athlete's bradycardia, a slower heart beat at rest because the heart is enlarged and stronger. An athlete's heart can be almost 50% larger than a normal heart and has enough to pump the blood around when it beats 40 to 50 beats per minute. That is not a problem. Not even when the athlete stops the sport. The heart then just gets a little bit smaller. The same as the impressive calf or glutes or biceps of a football player or a marathon runner which lose volume very fast if they break a leg and have to be immobilized for a little while. Also, age can make a difference from person to person. Some people have a resting heartbeat of 80 or 90 beats per minute and are really healthy.

It is also normal to feel an extrasystole once in a while, or an extra beat. Your heart is then beating too early and the pause until the next beat takes longer and therefore you have the impression that the heart is skipping a beat. Because the heart gets a little more time to fill with blood during the pause, the next beat is more forceful than normal. Extrasystole occur more often after the use of alcohol, coca cola, coffee, or chocolate, but also after exercise, strong emotions, or stress. People who suffer from extra heart beats can have that checked out even if it is only for their own peace of mind. Treatment is necessary if there are complaints associated with these extrasystole or if there are too many extrasystole which might increase the chance of getting heart failure.

Alarm signals and investigations

So what is then abnormal? People with a real rhythm problem or arrhythmia can feel all kinds of things or nothing at all. The symptoms vary from persistent palpitations and extrasystole to pain in the chest, shortness of breath, dizziness, hyperventilation, sweating, nausea, or the feeling that you can faint any second. These subjective feelings can be explained because the heart is beating too slow or too fast or too irregular and therefore it is inefficient and result in a lack of oxygen the body. We can explain it, but it is still frightening for the patient. There are quite a few people that feel with a rhythm problem fear they are having a heart attack when it happens for the first time, and that is good because then they are motivated to have it investigated straight away. We can investigate exactly what is happening by doing an ECG at rest or during a stress test. That is of course just a view at one particular moment, and you have to have a little bit of luck if just at that moment you have the arrhythmia. That is why in many cases we ask patients to have a 24-hour or 48-hour holter recording whereby we measure each heartbeat over that particular time frame. Another option is to do an electrophysiological investigation which happens in the hospital and is an invasive procedure where we measure the electrical system of the heart.

Treatment

Acute: People with an acute arrhythmia can often be treated with drugs that can prevent serious side effects like a stroke or a cardiac standstill, or drugs that restore the normal rhythm. Calcium antagonists keep calcium out of the heart muscle cell so that they contract less strongly. Beta blocking agents reduce the effect of stress hormones and lower the heart rhythm. Antiarrhythmics influence the electrical conduction from the heart rhythm from one cell to the other cell. Anticoagulation drugs will prevent thrombosis hence the lower risk of a stroke. Also, after the acute treatment people often require medication. When we have heart rhythms that go too fast and do not revert back to normal, we can do an electrical cardioversion. Cardioversion means to put the heart from one state into a normal state, so the Cardiologist who does the cardioversion is able to regain normal rhythm. This cardioversion is often used in case of atrial fibrillation. You are anaesthetised for a couple of minutes and the heart is subjected to an electrical shock with a defibrillator. It is a similar type of procedure used during a heart standstill. The difference between the defibrillation from a cardiac arrest is that this is a heart reset, while the electrical cardioversion in atrial fibrillation is synchronised to your normal rhythm.

Ablation

If drugs and cardioversion do not get the long-term result that is required, then ablation could be an option. Ablation is the destruction or removal of tissue but when we talk about rhythm abnormalities, we mean that we are neutralizing some tissue. During ablation, the doctor puts a catheter in the heart and the tip of the catheter can be very hot or very cold (cryoablation). This causes small scars and scar tissue does not conduct any electricity. The ablation can take place in different areas of the heart and that depends on where the rhythm abnormality originates from. Sometimes the doctor interferes with the area where the abnormal impulse starts, in other cases he inhibits an abnormal conduction pathway, or he insulates a certain route that the rhythm takes. So, let's have a look now at the most common arrhythmias.

14 ATRIAL FIBRILLATION

The most frequent cardiac arrhythmia is "atrial fibrillation" (AF). Other names you hear may be "atrial" or "supraventricular fibrillation". When you have atrial fibrillation, the rhythm of the atrial contraction is chaotic. On the ECG you do not find the little notch that normally occurs just before the high peak. Fibrillation means to thrill, and if the atria thrill instead of contracting together, then that can also influence the contraction of the ventricles. The ventricles during atrial fibrillation are usually still working well enough, approximately at 75% of their normal capacity. The real risk of atrial fibrillation is different. When you have this arrhythmia, the blood is not pumped efficiently in the chambers and stays in a part of the atrium going around like little whirlpools, and that can cause little blood clots. This usually happens in the left atrial appendage which is an appendage of the atrium that has a little niche and this niche usually helps the atria to pump the blood normally in the ventricle, but in case of atrial fibrillation it is an area where it is very easy for little blood clots to occur. These little blood clots can stay in the atrium but they can also move on, go into the left ventricle, and from the left ventricle in the body, and if that is by accident through an artery that leads to the brain then such a little blood clot can have very serious consequences. The atrial fibrillation enhances your chance of having a stroke or a heart attack and has to be treated always! At the time of the first atrial fibrillation the patient has to have medication immediately that aims to make the heart rhythm more regular and reduce the risk of developing a blood clot. If the drugs do not have the desired effect then atrial fibrillation can be solved in hospital with a cardioversion, but not all the time or only for a short period. The cardioversion has to be done within 48 hours of the start of the atrial fibrillation otherwise you have an increased risk that the shock will dislodge little blood clots. You can do cardioversion when the patient has been on anticoagulation medication for three weeks or longer or when the doctor does a transoesophageal guided cardioversion where he first looks with an ultrasound whether any blood clots are present in the atrium. Such a transoesophageal echocardiogram direct cardioversion is usually only done when it is urgent. In the case of young people with atrial fibrillation without significant heart abnormalities, ablation might be the best solution, especially if the occurrence of atrial fibrillation is intermittent. Often atrial fibrillation can be restored to a normal rhythm but sometimes it can't, or the problem will recur all the time.

If a patient does not prefer an operation/procedure or is not a candidate for this, then the doctor will prescribe medication which reduces the speed of the heartbeat. Atrial fibrillation occurs more often in the elderly and because our population is getting older, we will also see more of this. Every year the amount of people with atrial fibrillation is increasing. Only one to two percent of people younger than 65 will have atrial fibrillation. Except age, there are also other possible causes and risk factors. One is a thyroid gland which is working too hard, or being obese, a heart attack in the past, mitral valve leakage, high blood pressure—also temporarily high blood pressure because of nicotine or caffeine use, and alcohol misuse—especially binge drinking. Often there is not a clear cause and we call that idiopathic atrial fibrillation, or the phenomena are curtailed to only one occurrence of atrial fibrillation and we call that lone atrial fibrillation.

Atrial Flutter

If you have atrial flutter (to flutter means fast beating), the atria are contracting, in this case the atria are contracting together regularly but much too fast, approximately 300 times per minute. The node between the atrium and the ventricle, the AV node, can stop 50% of that exaggerated rate but then the ventricles are still contracting 150 times per minute at rest. On the ECG you see then a little saw tooth. Atrial flutter can change into atrial fibrillation. The risk factors and the treatment are approximately the same as with atrial fibrillation. Ablation seems to be very good treatment for this.

Sick sinus node

Sometimes the sinus node which is the built-in pacemaker of our heart is working too slowly, or not every sinus activation is being conducted though the tissue around it. We call this syndrome a "sick sinus node" or "sick sinus syndrome" (SSS—which is not a Holden!). Your heart is then beating too slowly for a healthy pump and the body is not getting enough blood. If your brain is suffering from lack of oxygen you can become unconscious, otherwise those symptoms are very similar as to when people suffer from atrial fibrillation. The cause of a SSS can also be another disease than one that has affected the sinus node itself, like obstructive sleep apnea or old age—the problem is a lot more prevalent in the elderly. Also medication given to prevent the heart beating too fast in the case of atrial fibrillation, for instance, can cause sick sinus syndrome. We can fix a sick sinus syndrome by replacing the natural pacemaker with an artificial pacemaker. If the heart is sometimes too fast and then by the same token too slow then the patient needs to receive a pacemaker to counteract the slow heart rate and medication to counteract the fast heart rate.

AV block

We are descending in the heart from the atria, the sinus node, and then to the AV node. An AV block you recall, is when the area between the atria and the ventricles cannot or only partially conduct the electrical impulse that arrives from the sinus node. The atrioventricular node is always slowing down the sinus node for just a moment because that is its function, but that will only be a fraction of a second. Possible causes of the AV block are wear-and-tear of the electrical conduction system, a heart attack, or the consequence of an operation or medication. The consequence of a partial or total AV block is that the ventricles will be too slow in contracting. They do contract but they are too slow. That is the reason why in cases of serious AV conduction abnormalities a pacemaker is implanted.

AVNRT

A disarranged AV node can also cause the heart to beat too fast. Often that happens through AVNRT which stands for "atrioventricular nodal re-entry tachycardia". It is a fast heartbeat because the impulse arrives into the AV node twice. When you have this problem (and we have multiple forms of this problem), there is in, or just adjacent to the normal AV node, an extra group of cells that together with the normal ones form a kind of circle, and that is why the impulse goes through the AV node to the ventricle but at the same time is circling around the roundabout in this extra group of cells resulting in a high heartbeat. This tachycardia is three times more prevalent in women than in men and we don't know exactly why. The problem can suddenly be apparent but also disappear again for years. Often it comes out of the blue. Other patients will tell you that alcohol or coffee can cause the racing, or it happens just after a short drop of blood pressure. If AVNRT is happening often, it is very inconvenient for the patient, but it is really not dangerous. Some people can deal with the problem themselves by pushing on their carotid artery but discuss this with your doctor before you start it, or to exhale and then keep your nose and mouth shut. This is the so-called Valsalva manoeuvre. Sometimes medications are necessary or an ablation whereby the doctor eliminates one of the two groups of cells that cause the arrhythmia. This carries the risk of course that the other group of cells is also attacked which means there is no conduction, you have a total AV block and then you do need a pacemaker.

Wolff-Parkinson-White

The WPW syndrome was described first by the American doctors Louis Wolff and Paul Dudley White and the Brit John Parkinson. WPW is very similar to the AVNRT, but you have to be careful not to confuse the two. Normally there is only one place in the isolating tissue between the atria and the ventricles where the sinus node activity can get through from the atrium to the ventricle, the so-called AV node. The AV node stops the signal momentarily and then allows the electrical activity to go via the bundle of His and the purkinje system to the ventricles, and this means that first the atria can contract together followed by all the blood pumped into the ventricles. When we talk about a WPW syndrome, there is an extra area separated from the bundle of His that can conduct the activity from the atrium to the ventricles. That extra bundle is called the bundle of Kent, so this is not a little circuit in the AV node as with AVNRT but really an alternative route that can be used by the electrical activity to go from atrium to ventricle. The difference is that when the electrical activity goes through the bundle of Kent, there is no break and there is no time, but the activity goes straight through from the atrium to the ventricle. That means that the ventricles are being activated too early and the heart rate is getting higher. Through this extra bundle of Kent, we can also observe the electricity going from ventricle back to the atrium, and then you can have a circuit whereby the rhythm is even further deranged. Where the bundle of Kent is exactly located is different in person to person. Sometimes it goes through the left atrium and sometimes it goes through the right atrium. You are born with it. On an ECG, you often see in case of a WPW a little nick in the left leg of the peak. The standard treatment is ablation. A little bit over 1 in 1000 people would have this abnormality, but we don't know this exactly. Often people have no symptoms so maybe there are more people that have it. Until the patient has arrhythmias, we don't know, and sometimes these arrhythmias cause the heart to stand still and death. That is rare, approximately four cases per thousand WPW's per year, but it does happen when the person had no knowledge of having a WPW before. Sometimes WPW syndrome causes rhythm abnormalities in young people, other people suffer from it later in life, and some people never. But like many things in cardiology, having those symptoms is something quite different than having a risk. WPW is a good example of that. Just like a lot of other cardiovascular submarines. People who are against preventive investigations for this kind of rare but possibly fatal condition often say that population screening is costing too much in comparison to the amount of life that can be saved if screening were to take place. That is a very harsh approach. It is logical that governments will have a budget and can focus on screening that will enable people to have as many healthy life years as possible. But still, I think the government has to do everything in their power to look at more rare conditions, especially when these conditions can have such a major impact on the individual that has the misfortune to be born with this.

Bundle branch block

We talk about bundle branch block when one of the two branches which divide the bundle of His are not conducting or badly conducting the electricity. The patient doesn't note this because the heart is just beating as normal, but you can see this abnormality on the ECG. A left bundle branch block is almost always a sign of an underlying heart problem and has to be evaluated. The status of the electrical system, the left ventricle and the coronary arteries have to be checked. A right bundle branch block is much more common and has usually no complaints and most of the time is benign. If there are complaints, then this block can be indicative of a malfunctioning right side of the heart possibly leading from a lung problem.

Ventricular fibrillation

The deadliest rhythm abnormality is ventricular fibrillation. In ventricular fibrillation, it is not the atria but the ventricles that move chaotically and lose their pump function completely. The only way to solve this problem is to apply an electric shock. Ventricular fibrillation is rare and seen much less than atrial fibrillation. It is almost always part of other heart problems and is usually the direct cause of sudden death. As high blood pressure is more a symptom or a risk factor than a real disease, so is ventricular fibrillation a result of the disease. People that survive ventricular fibrillation because they received cardiac massage, CPR and defibrillation outside the hospital are sometimes provided with an implantable cardioverter defibrillator or ICD. An ICD is a pacemaker that can not only manage slow heart rates but also fast heart rates and even ventricular fibrillation. When ventricular fibrillation is detected by the device it does exactly the same as an external defibrillator does, but inside the body. With an implanted ICD the heart can still have the fibrillation, but the ICD will shock the heart back into normal rhythm. However, you might lose consciousness, but then after a couple of seconds you regain consciousness because the device did its job. If you want to see how this happens, you can go to YouTube and look at Van Loo Hart. Here you will find a little film of a minute that shows the soccer player Antony Van Loo on the 9th June 2009 when he was playing soccer. At second 7, the 20-year-old player suddenly falls to the floor on his back. On second 14, you see how his body jumps and on second 20 he is sitting upright once again. He had an ICD implanted because he was diagnosed 12 months before with a serious rhythm abnormality. We have to remember though that the underlying heart condition is usually determined whether the patient will survive the ventricular fibrillation episode even when they have an ICD. Sometimes the heart is so damaged that the ventricular fibrillation will reoccur all the time and the treatment doesn't have any long-term success and the patient still dies.

Brugada Syndrome

The Brugada syndrome is a congenital disease of the heart whereby normal healthy-looking people get ventricular tachycardia or ventricular fibrillation and therefore suddenly lose consciousness or die. This especially happens at night. Fever and some medication can provoke the symptoms. There are probably multiple genetic mishaps or combinations that cause Brugada Syndrome, but one third of the patients suffer from mutation of the SCN5A-gene. That gene controls a protein which is of importance for the sodium pump through the cell wall and therefore also important for the contraction of the myocardial muscle cells. For heart contractions, you need electrical impulses, and so-called ions. The important ions are calcium, sodium, and potassium. In one in three patients with Brugada Syndrome, you find that there is not enough sodium in the heart muscle cells. Children of a mother or father with Brugada have a 50% risk of having the disease or the tendency to have the disease as well. You see Brugada Syndrome relatively seldom. According the European Commission's rare disease definition it is a disease that occurs in <5:10,000 people, and 1:2,000 people, but there are possibly more. The Brugada Syndrome is in any case the most important cause of SUDS or Sudden Unexplained Death Syndrome, which is the picture where people suddenly die without any obvious cause on autopsy. The Brugada Syndrome is responsible for 50% of all sudden death in people below the age of 40. In South East Asia, we find the syndrome much more often than anywhere else in the world. In Thailand and Laos, for instance, the Brugada Syndrome is, after traffic accidents, the most important cause of death in young males.

Twenty-five percent of all-natural death is caused by acute heart death. Scientists are looking into these phenomena, but it is not simple because the exact cause is usually not known and there are many possible causes that seem plausible. The Brugada Syndrome is only one of these causes. Another genetically manifested and potential deadly arrhythmia is the Long QT Syndrome, especially in children. You have also very rare forms like the Short QT Syndrome, especially in younger people; CPVT with children and ARVD/C which is especially known in young athletes. I am sure that in the years to come we will have more diseases and genetic factors that are related to sudden death. I was working in Maastricht, The Netherlands, when in 1986 Pedro Brugada first saw a Polish child of three years of age who came with his father because he had unexplained syncope and he had to reanimate his child. The electrocardiogram of this boy was very similar to that of his sister who died at the age of two, also after she had several episodes of syncope. This sister took medication and had a pacemaker which didn't help. These two children died from the same family which was the reason Pedro started his investigation and together with his two brothers, published the first articles which was then later coined by a Japanese Cardiologist "Brugada Syndrome". In 1992 they published eight patients who were revived after a cardiac arrest. The electrocardiograms showed a right bundle branch block and they linked this with the sudden death. The average age of these people was between 35 and 40 years. The youngest was at the time of death six months, the oldest 74. Further follow up and intensive investigations by many groups showed that this was caused by a genetic abnormality. The diagnosis can sometimes happen on a normal ECG but in many cases the typical abnormalities are not clear on the ECG and therefore you have to try and provoke the abnormalities with the use of drugs such as Ajmaline or Flecainide (=special drugs used in Cardiology). If the diagnosis is made, you can test the blood relatives with an ECG or provocation tests and then you can do further investigations like genetic testing. The treatment usually consists of an internal defibrillator, and that depends on the patient's specific risk. There is also a study going on to see whether ablation techniques can help in people with Brugada Syndrome. As a closure of this piece about Brugada Syndrome, we need to realise that some medications are dangerous for Brugada patients, and if you want to look into this more specifically look then on the internet under the heading brugadadrugs.org which is a very good website regarding this subject.

15 ABNORMALITIES AND DISEASE OF YOUR HEART MUSCLE OR CARDIOMYOPATHY

A cardiomyopathy is a chronic disease of the heart muscle itself. When the heart muscle is not able to contract or relax properly it means the pump function is not good, and the blood is not being pumped around the body properly. The disease is pretty common, but you have all different kinds of cardiomyopathies. You have a dilated cardiomyopathy (DCM) and a hypertrophic cardiomyopathy (HCM) which are most common. DCM is a disease whereby the muscle is floppier, and the heart is enlarged or dilated. That means that the pump is not strong anymore and especially when exercising cannot work or be able to meet the demand. The heart valves are also less effective because of this dilatation. In case of an HCM, part of the heart muscle is thickened, usually the piece of muscle between the left and the right ventricle. When the heart muscle is thickened it is not able to contract well, is less elastic, and therefore cannot pump as well. Sometimes in addition there is also a dilatation of one of the ventricles or both ventricles, another reason it cannot pump properly. The thickening can cause obstruction of outflow through the aortic valve and if that is the case, we call that obstructive HCM or HOCM (hypertrophic obstructive cardiomyopathy).

A pretty rare but very special disease is the Takotsubo cardiomyopathy or the broken heart syndrome. Takotsubo is a Japanese word for an octopus vessel, a ceramic vessel that fisherman use in Japan to catch octopus. When you have this disease, your left ventricle looks like such a pot. It was first described in Japan. Takotsubo not only causes extreme pain on the chest, but also the electrocardiogram makes you think the patient has a heart attack with ST segment elevation and so forth. When you investigate those people further in the hospital, you cannot find narrowing in the coronary arteries, but there is an abnormality in the bottom part of the left ventricle which makes it look like such a ceramic vessel. Normally the left ventricle has the form of an ice cream cone but with Takotsubo the bottom part of this cone swells up and looks like a balloon. On the outside of the heart you can't see it. It is the inner side, the cavity of the left ventricle, which becomes that way. It has as a consequence that the left ventricle does not pump well anymore. Women over 50 after menopause especially suffer from Takotsubo, sometimes because of an emotional crisis like a broken heart being in love, the death of a dear family member, or another situation of extreme emotional stress. Maybe it is related to the hormones that are being released under these emotions and have a negative influence on the heart muscle. Usually in most cases within a couple of weeks the abnormalities are reversed, and the patient feels a lot better, at least from a cardiac point of view.

Some cardiac muscle diseases have a genetic base. The direct cause is the ongoing stress on the heart muscle caused by an infection, high blood pressure, arrhythmias, narrowing of the coronary arteries, or diseases of the heart valve, but also diabetes, thyroid disease, alcoholism, being drug dependent, or important medical treatments like chemotherapy or radiation therapy can promote cardiomyopathies.

The complaints vary quite a bit from person to person and from time to time, but people usually complain about tiredness, shortness of breath, dizziness, getting out of bed to pass urine at night-time, or having an abnormal heartbeat. Sometimes the damage done on the heart muscle is reversible. The treatment is therefore treating the symptoms and preventing it from becoming worse. Patients have to rest, not drink alcohol, not get an infection, and sometimes the doctor will advise them to have certain drugs as well to stimulate the healing of the heart. If nothing is being done, then the next step would be that the heart is failing to work, and you might need then a heart transplant.

Cardiac failure

We have been discussing cardiac failure at some points in this book already, when the heart doesn't work properly as a result of many of the problems that we have discussed before. We call heart failure cardiac decompensation. Decompensation means that the heart is not able to fix its problems. Cardiac failure is chronic and serious because the pump function is reduced and usually the damage that caused this is irreversible. The degree of complaints is usually categorized in four categories depending on the type of exercise you can do. So this goes from just having complaints when you are doing a serious exercise or having complaints at normal exercise but not at rest, of having complaints at minimal exercise or even at rest. Also, the degree of cardiac failure is divided into two big brackets. The failure of the left ventricle which happens most often and failing of the right ventricle. Those two can happen together, but also separately. Often when the left ventricle fails over a long enough period of time the right ventricle is affected as well and you get biventricular heart failure. You have heart failure where the heart is not able to contract, but you also have heart failure where the heart is not able to relax properly. If the heart cannot relax properly it doesn't fill with enough blood each beat. When you have a reduction in pump function, it usually has to do with the left ventricular function. If you don't pump properly in the left ventricle the blood will stay there, or in the left atrium and you get congestion with elevated pressures in the lung and in the end in the right ventricle as well. So from this congestion the name congestive heart failure originates. Something similar happens when the right ventricle is not contracting properly. There is less blood going to the lungs and there is less blood that is getting oxygen, so you get the vicious cycle and because the heart is not pumping properly, the lungs are not working properly, there is less oxygen in the blood, the organs don't function properly because they are not getting enough oxygen and nutrients. But even if the ventricles can contract properly but not relax properly, you still have cardiac failure. This is caused because in between the contraction, the heart cannot relax enough and when it is not relaxed it cannot receive enough blood, so during each heartbeat not enough blood can be pumped around. In the end you get the same consequences as with predominantly left-sided cardiac failure. You will feel tired, you get fluid in the lungs which is pulmonary oedema, and the body that is programmed to sustain itself will try to compensate all these things and hence people can pedal along for a while before they crash.

There are many causes of cardiac failure. It could be the wear and tear of the body when we are get older, or we have early wear and tear because of the occurrence of high blood pressure and narrowing of the arteries, heart attacks, valve abnormalities, infections, rhythm abnormalities, abnormalities we are born with, and intrinsic diseases of the heart muscle itself. What we have left out so far is haemochromatosis which is a genetic abnormality in your iron household. This manifests in the accumulation of too much iron in different organs, also muscles like in the heart. The diagnosis is often missed and can only be confirmed with a liver biopsy or DNA investigations, but if the diagnosis is made, treatment is usually possible. Next to all the complaints that I just mentioned, people with cardiac failure often collect fluid as a consequence of the blood vessels that are very full and therefore start to leak. That is why their ankles and legs swell up, they have difficulty sleeping, and have to get out of bed at night often to pass urine. The treatment cannot reverse the damage done all the time, but the treatment can stabilize or slow down the process.

A leaking heart valve can be replaced or repaired, a narrowing in the arteries can be dilated with a balloon and a stent, and a rhythm abnormality can be solved with a pacemaker or ablation. With diuretics we can reduce the chance of getting oedema and we have different medications that reduce the risk of complications associated with cardiac failure. When people are discharged from hospital after an episode of cardiac failure, they usually get the advice to change their lifestyle: Not to drink too much fluid (restricted to between one and two litres), no alcohol at all, reduction of salt intake, no smoking, avoid heavy exercise but have regular exercises over the day, don't go to rides in Luna Park like a roller coaster, and so forth. The prognosis usually depends on which phase the cardiac failure presented itself and although you cannot cure it completely, if the reduction in function is not too bad and with the right medication and lifestyle changes, many people can have a relatively comfortable life.

There are too many patients, however, who are still blind to their symptoms and don't take the advice of their GP or Cardiologist and don't change their lifestyle or take the advice to have open heart surgery. Those people are usually not "difficult", but they are just afraid. They are afraid to change their habits, they are afraid to not have enough willpower to manage changes, they are afraid for the possible side effects of the medications, they are afraid for the risk of operations, they are afraid for not leaving the hospital alive, but if they don't then their life does not change from day to day, it just gets worse from day to day, and they have to accept that every day they are able to do a little bit less and that the quality of their life is going downwards. So they can stay at home, they can read, they can watch television, they can chat with their family, and enjoy a birthday party with the kids or the grandkids because maybe it is the last time.

If you have cardiac failure, for instance, because of a leaking heart valve, and you don't want an operation then over the years that problem will come so bad that your general condition will not allow any more surgery. You have to be admitted and re-admitted, and in the end, you are not going to leave the hospital. You get some oxygen, they can get some fluid out of your chest, they will give you some morphine, but the end is then and there. Yes, we do have to die of something, all of us, however there are a lot of factors that we ourselves can influence to determine the time and the circumstances in which we leave this earth. I do trust and hope that people reading this book will have the inspiration to keep themselves as fit and healthy as possible for a long time to come. Preventative care is important!

Cardiac transplants

Sometimes the condition of a human heart is that bad that only a new heart can solve the problem. A cardiac transplant is unfortunately not something that will happen for everybody that needs it. For starters, your heart failure has to be maximally treated without the desired result, and your changes to stay alive without the transplant would be minimal. There have to be no other problems that would jeopardize a new heart and you have to be fit enough to be able to take an operation like that. All these matters are extensively investigated and if you are going to be a candidate for cardiac transplant then of course they have to find a heart that is compatible with your body. There are not enough donor hearts and there are people dying every day on the waiting list. Part of the reason why we don't have that many donor hearts is because we are getting better in preventing car accidents which is in a way very good, but it means that the waiting time on a transplant list is unsure and not predictable. Sometimes there is a new heart a day after you are on the list, but some people have to perhaps wait two years or longer. Your Cardiologist cannot do anything about that. He will have the data about your heart and the organization that looks at all the criteria of all the people on the waiting list will in the end make the decision on who gets which heart. People who are on the transplant list are living difficult times, they have to be available on a permanent basis and have to be able to get into the hospital within a reasonable timeframe to have the transplant organized. In Western Australia, it means that people usually have to move into the city to live. During the period on the list, the candidate has to have regular medical check-ups, they have to live as healthily as possible, and avoid infections by staying out of the way of people who have a problem, and they also need to take immunizations because if you have another disease on top of your congestive heart failure you might not get your transplant. Some of the people on the transplant list are also a candidate for an artificial heart or an additional pump that is a bridge to a transplant. The extra mechanical pump can help to support your own heart and can be a bridge to the actual transplant. There is some research going on to give people a permanent additional heart, so they have their own heart and a mechanical heart implanted and this seems to be very promising but is still in the experimental stages.

When you do get a cardiac transplant your operation usually takes between four to six hours. Three weeks after this you are well enough to go home but you have to take multiple medications and have regular follow-ups for the rest of your life, even though the check-ups will be on a yearly basis in the end if everything goes okay. There are not that many transplants in Australia, but one of the reasons is that the treatment of congestive heart failure improves with new medication and alternative treatments. Also, the survival rate after cardiac transplant is increasing. In most centres in the world, 90% of the people who receive a transplant are alive after five years, and after ten years 75% of the patients are still alive. For them, a completely new chapter in their life has started. Most of the patients experience a spectacular improvement in their quality of life, they are stimulated to live healthily, and also to restart activities like going back to work, exercise, mountaineering, and so forth!

16 CONGENITAL ABNORMALITIES— SOMETHING YOU ARE BORN WITH

A little bit less than 1% of all babies are born with a heart abnormality. Heart abnormalities are therefore the most important form of a congenital abnormality. One out of 10 abnormal genetics have to do with the heart. Often the cause is genetics, but sometimes it is because during pregnancy something happened. A lot of serious abnormalities can be detected during pregnancy with the help of ultrasound. Sometimes they can only find it when the baby has been born, and sometimes years after birth. Also, the seriousness of the disease is quite different. Only mild abnormalities do not give any symptoms, other abnormalities require immediate surgery. The most common abnormalities are a little hole in between the right and the left ventricle called a ventricular septal defect (VSD). Because the blood pressure in the left side of the heart is higher than in the right side, usually there is oxygen rich blood going from the left ventricle to the right ventricle, so there is extra blood going to the lungs and that can cause a high blood pressure in the lungs. Babies with a VSD are often treated with a diuretic to make sure that not too much fluid is getting into the lung. Depending on the seriousness of the high blood pressure in the lung, a surgical procedure can be needed to close the little hole between the two ventricles. One out of 1500 babies born alive have an ASD which is a little hole in between the atria. Often the ASD is a consequence of a foramen ovale which stayed open. The foramen ovale is a normal opening between the two atria when the baby is still in the mother's womb and not needing their lungs. It enables the baby's body to have the blood that is being oxygenated via the placenta to get the blood from the left to the right side of the blood circulation. Normally this foramen ovale closes at the time of birth by itself. You don't always have to treat ASD's. If they are smaller than 3mm it does not mean that it has to be treated because it does not over stress the heart. Even bigger ones often still close themselves during the first 18 months. Children with a serious ASD have symptoms, they can be more easily tired or more often feel sick, and their development is slower, just as with a VSD. If an ASD is not spontaneously closing, we can close it with a catheter and a little umbrella device. When the ASD or VSD is fixed, children usually have a normal life expectancy, and they are able to do all kinds of exercises and activities other kids of their age can do. There are also many adults that have a little hole in the heart without knowing or having complaints.

Another opening which is normal when the baby is still in the womb is a connection between the pulmonary artery and the aorta. If that is not closed immediately after the birth, then we talk about an open ductus arteriosus. We find this more often in girls than in boys and often after the mother has suffered a rubella infection. With an open ductus arteriosus, too much blood goes through the lungs and so the heart can be over stressed. Sometimes, usually in babies which are born prematurely, the problem can be solved with medication. In other cases, the opening has to be plugged with the help of a catheter. One out of ten heart abnormalities that babies are born with has an intriguing name—the Tetralogy of Fallot which is a combination of four construction mishaps. One, a ventricular septal defect. Two, an aorta which is out of sync and is connected to both the right and the left ventricle. Three is a narrowing of the pulmonary artery valve and the fourth is a thickening of the right ventricular wall. Because of this combination the heart does not pump properly, but depending on how serious the construction defect is, the symptoms can be quite different from one child to another. Usually an operation is needed. The situation of the child improves quite a bit after the surgery, but it will need lifelong medical follow-up to be on top of possible complications that can occur later in life. Other congenital heart abnormalities are a narrowing of the aorta, a narrowing of a valve, or transposition of the big blood vessels. The last one is rare but very serious—the aorta is connected to the right ventricle and the pulmonary arteries on the left ventricle. The problem is that in this case there is no oxygen going from the lungs to the tissue of the organs. In utero it is not a problem because the baby gets the oxygen from the mother, but after the delivery, the baby has to be operated on straight away.

Cerebrovascular accident or CVA

CVA's are treated by a neurologist, but because they have to do with our blood circulation and because they are very common and because so much emphasis is placed on the early recognition of the problem, we will discuss it here briefly as well. When you have a CVA, part of the brain has lacked oxygen for some time. There are two kinds of CVA's—there is a brain infarct and there is a brain bleed. Most of the CVA's, probably eight out of ten, are infarcts. In this case, the same phenomena happen as with a heart attack. You get a brain attack; a little blood clot closes off a blood vessel and the area of the brain that depends on the blood supply from this blood vessel is in stress and might die. A brain bleed is when a blood vessel in the brain is damaged and starts to bleed. There is also a lighter and more temporal form of a CVA, a so-called transient ischaemic attack (TIA) or an episode of lack of oxygen which is only temporary. This is not always recognized and is a shame because a TIA or a mini stroke can be the messenger for a real stroke. The risk of a stroke can be calculated with a so-called CHADSVASc score. The formula seems difficult but not if you know what it stands for. The C stands for congestive heart failure or a left ventricle that doesn't work properly. The H stands for hypertension. The first A for age or, in particular, an age of 75 years or more. The D for diabetes and the S for stroke, whether the patient had one before. The V is for vascular disease like peripheral vascular disease or a heart attack in the past, angina pectoris, or atherosclerosis of the aorta. The second A is for an age between 65 and 75, and Sc is for sex category i.e. male or female. If one of those factors is applicable for yourself, then you get one point, except for the fact of 75 years or more and stroke—they are more serious and therefore you get two points for them. The higher the score, the higher the risk of a stroke. The maximum is 9 and not 10 because you are only in one of the two age categories, which is similar to an average stroke risk of 15.2% per year. The medication that you will receive depends on your score. If you have a score of zero, then anticoagulation (blood thinners) are probably not necessary. If you have a score of one or more, you will get them, and which one depends on your doctor and the patient. This means that different co-morbidities are taken into account to decide which anticoagulation drug or method is going to be used.

We know that in the days and hours before a heart attack people often have signs, although they are not always recognized, but usually most of the CVA's are completely out of the blue. The most important three symptoms that we recognize from a CVA is an abnormal mouth with sagging, a slurred speech, and a problem in an arm not being able to move properly, and those three items can occur together or each separately. If one of those things happen to you or somebody else, then immediately call an ambulance. It is important that if you are alone and you have a stroke and you can't speak, you still have to try to call the ambulance. Even if you can't speak people on the other side might figure out what is happening to you. There are other signs where part of the body doesn't work because the associated brain function is "temporarily not available", but they are not that often. People can have a weak leg, they can see double, or they can see only half the image or nothing at all, sudden dizziness, and in case of a brain bleed very severe headache for which you have no explanation. If you have one of these symptoms, the same recipe—call an ambulance. To never hesitate and call the ambulance straight away is very important because the first hours after a CVA are crucial to save as much brain tissue as possible. When you arrive in hospital, the doctor will see whether you really had a stroke, and they do that with a CT scan or MRI. If you have an infarct which has been less than four or five hours old, then you can often get treatment with thrombolysis. You will get an infusion with a drug that will thin the blood and clean up the blood clot in your brain. Within six hours, it can also sometimes be removed with the help of a catheter. The quicker the problem is solved, the bigger the chance you can have a good recovery. With a brain bleed the prognosis is usually not as good but it really depends on the size of the bleed. Sometimes an operation is necessary to prevent a new bleed. When the blood vessels in the brain are too wide or aneurysmatic, they can put in a little coil though a catheter which means that the aneurysm cannot burst. The surgeon can also surgically fix a dilatation of the blood vessels with a clip and there are several other ways to deal with the problem. A CVA can have many different results, in some people you don't notice a thing but in other people they need to learn everything again—it is like they are babies. Usually patients will have the most success with rehabilitation in the first six months when they start it. But there are some patients who years after their CVA and against all odds still improve. Our brains are obviously much more placid than we think!

17 INVESTIGATIONS OF THE HEART AND BLOOD VESSELS

You ain't seen nothing yet

I am a born optimist. The fact that every year almost 18 million people die because of heart or vascular disease does not mean that the average life expectancy in the last 100 years has decreased enormously, especially in the western countries. It is actually the other way around, it is because we live longer, that we have so many people with cardiovascular disease. A hundred years ago, the average life expectancy in the industrialised world was between 45 to 50 years. That was mainly because of the high death in children, but now the life expectancy is over 85 years of age. That is more than 50% increase. If it is going this way, then by the end of the 21st century we will be living until 130 years or more. That really sounds incredible today, but such an increase is not less likely now as it was 100 years ago. Au contraire that the life expectancy last century made such a big improvement but was done despite two world wars and all the problems we have had with a young, ever changing consumption society. The traffic accidents, the stress, the addictions, the unhealthy lifestyles, obesity, social isolation, depression, and our not taking care of the environment.

Today we are much more aware of all those unwanted side effects and our post-modern society tries to build in all the advantages whilst counteracting all the excess. This will only mean that the average age will increase even further. Thanks to technologies, law, dedication, and living standards in general, the working standards, and the way we organise our life, causes less accidents and less incidences. Our nutrition is better, our transport means are safer, and our hygiene is better (thanks COVID-19!). Since the 20th century, even something as trivial as the invention of a fridge has saved a lot of people dying from food poisoning. We are also much better in counteracting national disasters or pandemics or epidemics. We can't stop it, but we can predict them better, we can trace them better, and we can take worldwide appropriate measures to minimise the damage. You wouldn't say so if you watched the news every day because the news is more focused on the exception than the rule, but it is getting better every day with the people over the whole world and that is the trend. If only we could do something meaningful about climate change, the disparity in income, the violence related to religion, the overpopulation of the earth, and the management of armed conflict in that case, and then we would have as humankind a beautiful future. And for those people who long for the days of yesterday, think about all the graveyards full of dead children and the time that when you turn 100 years you were in the newspaper, now it is the other way around. Every 13 years we have twice as many people living over 100 years of age.

The most important factor for this particular rise in average age is our medical know-how and what we are able to provide for our community. We have more and ever better vaccines, medical drugs, medical instrumentation, operation techniques, methods in tracing disease, imaging, data banks, ambulances, hospitals, and even better trained researchers by medical scientists, doctors, and nurses. There are quite a few people that fear we are done with medicine and medical scientific improvements and that there are no big leaps to be expected. Well that is fortunately not right. Medical science is not a science that looks into a forest and only that forest. Science is something that looks into the whole universe in all types of dimensions. Just like astronomers look further and further into the universe, and molecular biologists and quantum physics look deeper and deeper into very, very, very small units of life. Every door that science can open, has access to a corridor with new doors. There is so much still to explore and discover. From your brain only a fraction is known. The importance of the microbiome in your gut, the billions of bacteria and the hundreds of different types in our colon, we don't realise it yet, but human genetics is also a big mystery for the most part. We know about genes and gene mutations, but we don't know the exact effects on them and change in them.

A good part of our medical advantages is related closely to the miniaturisation of computer chips. Every time we think we have the ultimate chip or the miniscule camera invented, engineers are coming up with a version which is again more powerful and smaller. There is a lot happening at the present with integration of digital technology in people and other biological symptoms. The possibilities in the field of cybernetics, nanotechnology, bionic implants, and gene technology, are unbelievable. Self-learning computers and robots are looking more and more like humans, but the reverse is true too, it is not impossible that our brain one day will manage our arms and legs without the use of the spine, or it is not unthinkable that we can deal with external data banks just by thinking about it. We can already make new tissue or fix damaged tissue outside the body as well as inside the body. Better than ever before we can understand diseases, we can prevent diseases, we can cure diseases, we can manage diseases, and we can find them and diagnose them much earlier because of a wide arsenal of investigation methods. In the last years, medical imaging techniques are so improved that doctors can study the human body with more precision and with less risk or negative effects for the patients from the outside, or with minute cameras from the inside. Scientists are working at present to make echocardiography devices which are 50x better than the current ones and MRI techniques which can show a beating heart in miniscule detail. Another important evolution is the development of the so-called wearables which are sensors that you can wear and that measure parameters like your heart beat, your blood pressure, your body temperature, your stress level, and sometimes also your potassium levels, your sugar levels, and so forth. With these types of techniques, a patient can be monitored for a long time and it can be used to send a signal if there is a problem. Scientists are trying to develop wearable systems that warn patients when they should see the doctor, even before they have one single symptom. In health care in the future, we will have chips in wrist bands, in plasters on your skin, implant devices, or swallowable cameras which constantly look at us and see whether anything changes causing a deleterious effect. The big data that is found like this will be collected by applications and super-computers full of fancy algorithms. They will filter and analyse all this data, and patients and/or their doctor will be automatically wire-lessly communicated when it is time to investigate further or to inter-vene. So if people think that this is the end of our evolution, nope; we ain't seen nothing yet. Even today when we read this, the investigation methods to look for cardiovascular problems is impressive.

I hope that the reader does not have heart or vascular disease, but if you do then there was never a better time to get it as now. What we are talking about here is how you and I can find out whether there is a heart problem. We will start with the most simple and cheapest way of investigation and after which we look at more complex, more expensive, and more invasive techniques.

Everything starts with a good chat

The first investigation has nothing to do with technology, at least not the technology we were thinking about just now. It is related to the chat you have with your GP, that discussion is the basis for the diagnosis and treatment. You are asked to mention or describe as well as possible, your complaints. Maybe you had chest pain, maybe you had palpitations, maybe you were short of breath or dizzy or maybe you had some swelling of your ankles or pain in your legs, maybe you have to get out of bed at night to pass urine, maybe you feel a lack of energy, maybe you have to cough a lot. It could also be that you have no specific complaints and that you are unsure whether you have any cardiovascular problem. In both cases the doctor will ask you questions about risk factors like your weight, how much you move, whether you smoke, whether you have high blood pressure. If he is your general doctor that you see regularly, then he knows which medication you are using, but that is also discussed. You can expect questions regarding heart and vascular disease in the family or relatives who died young from a heart attack, for instance. Maybe you have a genetic predisposition for heart disease. It is also up to you to ask questions yourself. Talking to your doctor is also a spontaneous way of saying things that perhaps could be important. A good chat is really necessary because dealing with the heart or vascular disease is not a one stop shop and it is important to have regular discussions with your GP about these issues.

After the history, it is time to do the first physical examination. They measure your blood pressure, listen to your heart and lungs, and check whether your body shows any outside signs of heart disease or issues that could be associated with increased risk to have or to get heart disease, like and abnormal colour of your skin or accumulation of fluid somewhere. They might even perform an ECG, and if your doctor thinks it is necessary, he might refer you to a Cardiologist. A

Cardiologist can do some additional tests like a stress test or an echocardiogram, and in hospital they have even more options to check you out.

Second opinion?

Perhaps your first contact is really your second or maybe even your third contact because you wanted a second opinion. To want a second opinion can be due to multiple reasons, maybe you are not convinced or maybe you just don't have a good bond with your doctor. You think he is too old, or she is too young, or you found on the internet information that is not the same as what your doctor is telling you.

Maybe you have a dilemma? Perhaps you are thinking, 'I want to do everything to check out my concern but the risk that I put a strain on the relationship with my doctor is maybe bigger. I don't want to seem to be a nut case.' I think that it is important that if you are not sure about the diagnosis or the way that your doctor deals with a problem, then it is a very good idea to ask the opinion of a different doctor. I think that in general, doctors have less problems with asking for second opinions or have people come in for a second opinion or people going away for a second opinion than patients. You should also not be afraid to discuss your questions or your considerations or your dilemma with your doctor. If your doctor understands his profession and what he is supposed to do as your doctor, he will be very positive and use this opportunity to give you extra explanation why he thinks in a certain way and why he gives you this particular advice. If that is not good enough for you then he will not hesitate to refer you to somebody else for a second opinion. I think he should also co-operate by giving the other doctor all the information he has gathered already so that you don't have to do double investigations. It is also possible that your doctor will discourage you from getting a second opinion if he thinks that is not in your benefit, but he will have the opportunity then to explain to you why he thinks it is not a good idea. Maybe your disease is urgent, and you cannot wait for your second opinion. If you feel that your doctor is not reacting appropriately or is not polite or friendly, then probably you have the wrong doctor anyway and you are better off to get another one. If you talk to your doctor and be honest with him, you can never go wrong. If the relationship is not okay then, you have no problem in finding another one and you never have the feeling that you did something behind somebody's back.

A second and even a third opinion is sometimes helpful because, if anything, it will clarify the issues around your disease problem. There might not be a clear-cut answer or treatment, but you will benefit from understanding the line of thought and the relationship with your doctor will improve. This is important because if you both decide to go down a certain path of diagnosis and treatment, then you have the best chance that you will finish that journey and come out the other side a much healthier person. If you do go for a second or third opinion, it is not necessary to stay with that particular doctor, you get their advice and then choose the doctor that is best for you. I think you should be careful with "medical shopping", because at some point in time you have to accept that there are different opinions and different visions on how to get to a certain point. You must make a decision and go with one. It is important that you allow a certain strategy time to actually work for you and that you clearly understand what the advantages and the disadvantages of the treatment are, and that the advantages are more significant than the disadvantages. A plan of treatment always needs to be evaluated and re-evaluated, at which point alterations or change of treatment can be discussed. That is why it is important that you have a good relationship with your doctor.

Doctors are human beings and therefore they can be wrong. It is a pity and sometimes dangerous though if a treatment does not have the desired effect because the patient did not give it the appropriate chance. Also consider that a second or third opinion costs more time and you are losing time which can sometimes be important. It is also true that if doctors come to the conclusion that they can't help or don't know what the best mode of action is, they will ask you to go for a second opinion to a colleague of theirs more specialised in that particular problem, and definitely if we are going to talk about decisions like euthanasia or patients who are at risk of suicide.

Auscultation of the heart

We listen to the heart with a stethoscope. The technique of listening to the heart is very old but a trained ear of the doctor can still hear a lot about the function of the heart. Heart auscultation is very important in the first encounter with the patient. The stethoscope is nothing else than a big ear drum with a tube, ear plugs, and a funny name. "Stethos" is a Greek word for chest, but "scope" refers to looking. A stethophone would be much more logic because the doctor is listening not looking at specific points on your chest, just on top of specific parts of the heart, but also at some parts in the armpit, neck, and back. He is listening to the heartbeat, the two heart tones which are produced by the closing of the heart valves. The first tone is produced by the mitral and tricuspid valve and the second heart tone is caused by the closing of the aortic and pulmonary valve. Sometimes these tones are split, or they are too mumbled or there are too many tones. In young people and pregnant women, often a third heart tone is normal, but it can also be a sign of heart failure. A fourth heart tone can be caused by thickening of the ventricular wall. Apart from the tone, the doctor can also evaluate the speed and regularity of the heartbeat or he can be looking for different beats and sounds. A heart murmur can be innocent but in adults also it can be related to a narrowed heart valve. When the murmur is occurring during the heart cycle is important, how loud it is, at what spot is the loudest, and whether you can hear it elsewhere in the chest or even sometimes on the head (I wrote about that in 1984; Het Kukelfenomeen and Ned Tijdschr Geneeskd 1984;128:nr26). Sometimes you can hear a shrieking noise which could be caused by pericarditis, an inflammation of the little tissue sac around the heart muscle itself.

18 MEASURING YOUR BLOOD PRESSURE (KEEP YOUR BLOOD PRESSURE DOWN*)

The classic way to measure blood pressure is as follows—the doctor puts a tourniquet around the upper arm and pumps it up with a little gummy pear-like device which causes the blood flow through the arm to reduce every time he pumps the pressure up. The doctor puts pressure against the pressure that the heart uses to pump the blood through the arm to your fingers. During the blood pressure measurement, the doctor feels your pulse. After a couple of pumping actions of the gummy pear the tourniquet presses hard on the artery in the arm so that the pulse felt by the doctor is gone. The measuring device, the manometer, now gives the maximal blood pressure. It reflects the maximal blood pressure just at a time that the heart is contracting. The doctor checks this by pumping the tourniquet up a little bit further and, after that, slowly releasing the pressure while he or she is listening with the stethoscope on the inner side of the elbow to listen to the blood flow through the artery. At a certain moment, he hears certain tones, the so-called Korotkoff tones, and he will then again look at what the values are. The pressure that he finds has to be very similar to the first valve he found, which was the upper pressure, the so-called systolic pressure. Subsequently he lets go of more pressure by releasing the tourniquet until all the Korotkoff tones have disappeared, and that is the moment the device will measure the lower pressure, the so-called diastolic blood pressure. The unit of blood pressure is "millimeters of mercury" and this reflects back to the times we used a mercury manometer and was related to the elevation of the mercury under the influence of the blood pressure being read when the mercury is put in a thin glass column. This technique was invented at the end of the 19th century by an Italian paediatric doctor Scipione Riva-Rocci: that is why we still use the letters RR when we refer to blood pressure measurements. In some places we now leave the RR and just call it BP.

24-hour BP monitoring

Blood pressure is variable: during the day it is usually higher than at night and is also higher when you do exercise, when you are emotional, and sometimes also when you have to go and see the doctor—the famous "white coat syndrome". To get a more realistic picture about blood pressure, it can be valuable to measure the blood pressure during a longer period of time than only the single moment you are visiting the doctor. For a 24-hour blood pressure measurement device, you will have a tourniquet around your arm with a little blood pressure device that you wear with a belt around your hip. You can take the belt off at night, but you have to keep the tourniquet on. The device measures your heartbeat and your blood pressure automatically a couple of times per hour during the day and at night, but at night usually less often. The device is fully automatic and has a memory for all the measurements taken. The patient is supposedly doing his normal daily activity except for making the device wet. Most devices do not tolerate water so you cannot take a shower, have a bath, or go for a swim. When you have your measurement, you are required to keep your arm still at that particular point of time. You can also keep a diary from that day and especially when you are emotional or when you are taking your medications.

A very good alternative for this 24-hour blood pressure measurement device is buying your own blood pressure machine which is not that expensive. You measure your blood pressure every time you wake up in the morning and when you go to bed. This can also give the doctor a pretty good idea what the variations are in your blood pressure and help with to determine whether you do have high blood pressure or not and, if you do, what type of treatments would be the best suitable and whether they are working.

Measurement of blood pressure yourself is getting more and more common and it is clear nowadays that this method works better as a strategy to prevent cardiovascular risks than just when people in health care centres measure your blood pressure. Even though the measurement might not be perfect, it is very good when people measure their own blood pressure because the "white coat syndrome" effect is usually not there and the blood pressure is measured multiple times over many days or weeks which gives a much better indication about the realistic blood pressure. The other reason it is important is that people who measure their own blood pressure are usually more aware of their health and they are more motivated to deal with their risk factors. Measuring your blood pressure is especially useful for people who are at high risk, i.e. people who are over the age of 50, people with diabetes, pregnant women, possible high blood pressure patients, and diagnosed high blood pressure patients. When you measure your own blood pressure you are probably better off buying a blood pressure machine with a tourniquet for the upper arm as they are much more sensitive and reliable than the ones that use the pulse or finger. But technology is moving fast so these devices will improve greatly over the next couple of years. If you are not too sure about which device to buy, you can always ask the advice of the pharmacist or your GP. Measuring blood pressure is best done when you are sitting with your feet on the floor after five minutes of rest without talking or moving, before having food or at least three hours afterwards. If you take antihypertensive medication and if you do not have any high blood pressure according to the measurements at home, then do not stop your blood pressure medication but use these measurements to discuss with your Cardiologist or GP. After all, you might have a low blood pressure because you are taking this medication! (* Instagram: Heartcare_by_Dr_Janssen)

Blood investigations—the lab work!

You can make a correlation with engine oil and the state of the engine as your blood is about your heart and your body. To take some blood the doctor or the nurse puts a little tourniquet around your arm so that the veins are a little bit dilated and more easily accessible for the needle. Usually the little needle is connected to a plastic tube that goes into a collection tube. It is rare but sometimes it is necessary to fast before you have your blood test. Usually the doctor who requests the blood test will tell you whether you need to be fasting. Fasting means no water, tea, or coffee at least two hours before the bloodletting and at least six hours before, no other drinks, meals, or milk products, and at least eight hours before the bloodletting no other food. The doctor usually gives you a form on which he jots down what he would like to test and then the laboratory will bring the blood samples to the lab and get it tested. In people with cardiovascular disease they will usually test your different cholesterol levels like your HDL, your LDL, your triglycerides, and depending on whether you see your doctor for the first time or whether it is a follow up. he might want to check specific things like the stress hormone of the heart, your iron levels, some hormones, some vitamins, and so forth. He might also do a blood test to check whether the blood thinning medication you might be using is working correctly. An important part of the blood tests are constructing a risk profile for you, and this might include items like your sugar levels, your kidney function, your heart enzymes like your troponin, and sometimes even more fancier stuff like growth hormone, calcium levels, phosphate levels, vitamin levels—like vitamin D, vitamin C, vitamin B12, and so forth. The doctor will explain to you why he thinks he will need certain information and discuss the results with you.

With the blood investigations of your cardiac enzymes like your troponin, AST, LDH, CK, the doctor can check whether you have had a heart attack or having a heart attack. When you suffer from a myocardial infarction or a heart attack, cardiac cells are damaged and that causes certain enzymes to be released, so-called cardiac enzymes. The more serious the heart attack the more cardiac enzymes are found in the blood, so people find that your creatinine kinase—your CK, your lactate dehydrogenase—your LDH, and your troponin, might be elevated. This last one, the troponin, is definitely elevated six hours after a heart attack and you can find it up to two weeks after a heart attack in blood samples.

Measuring the sugar and diabetes

It is often after an investigation for possible heart problems or blood vessel problems that people are suddenly made aware that they have diabetes. Often, they do not have any symptoms of diabetes and the diagnosis is only made because the doctor is not only measuring the cholesterol and triglycerides, but also the sugar levels. Type 2 diabetes is often associated with high blood pressure, obesity, and a higher cholesterol levels—a cocktail which will increase your cardiovascular risk considerably. Patients who have this diagnosis have an important task ahead in getting good medical care and follow up.

Being afraid of blood: fainting!

Some people, even some doctors, are very afraid to have their blood taken. They get a funny feeling in the stomach, a cold sweat is pouring out, and they really have to stay focused to not faint. In medicine we call this a "vasovagal syncope", which is losing consciousness as a result of a sudden drop in blood pressure by over activity of the tense brain nerve, the so-called nervus vagus. Your brain then gets just a little bit less oxygen for a moment and you faint. Other possible causes are standing up for a long time, hunger, over-exhaustion, or a hit on your plexus solaris which is a nerve knot between your belly button and your breastbone. Because you fall when you faint, you land in a horizontal position which allows blood to go to your brain and you will regain consciousness all by yourself. So that is the reason why when you have a blood test, they will put you horizontal on the table if you mention that you suffer from fainting. The bloodletting is not painful, the little sting is only a split second and disappears very quickly. It is watching the blood flow that most people don't like. One in seven people that have their blood taken have a blood pressure drop by seeing the blood. This could be an evolution thing.

Neanderthals who were wounded during fights and had the genetic variant to lose consciousness by looking at blood would fall down, seeming to be dead. They were left alone by their enemies and because their blood pressure was low, they didn't lose as much blood than otherwise. This way they had a better chance to survive and to give their genetic variant to their offspring. As we have become more professional and use much more deadly weapons like bullets and bombs instead of arrows, spears, and swords, the fainting gene was less relevant. Whoever has it today just finds it a nuisance. But it can also be that this blood phobia has nothing to do with genetics, but more to traumatic experiences during childhood. Other than looking away during the bloodletting procedure and talking about something else with the person who is doing it, there is nothing else you can do.

There are training programs whereby you are taught to first increase your blood pressure by increasing the tension in your muscles and psychology training by imagining that you go the doctor and that they are taking your blood by looking at movies, seeing a needle being prepared, etc.

The electrocardiogram or ECG

An electrocardiogram or ECG or EKG registers the electrical activity of the heart muscle. The device that they use to measure this is called the ECG machine or electrocardiograph. The Dutch doctor Wilhelm Einthoven who invented the device was awarded a Nobel Prize for medicine in 1924 for this. On an ECG you can measure the speed and the regularity of the heart rate and it is diagnostic for some diseases. You can see some heart rhythm abnormalities whether the heart has lack of oxygen, an acute myocardial infarction, an older myocardial infarction, or an enlarged heart. You cannot see whether the heart is pumping well directly on an ECG.

An ECG works with electrodes that are placed on the skin. The electrical activity of the heart is not measured on the heart itself usually, but sometimes during open heart surgery. The electrodes on the skin pick up the current that is leaking from the heart to the skin. You don't feel it, so you are not aware of it. That current is therefore also very small, only a few millivolts, which are thousandths of a volt. The person who is being investigated with the ECG has to lay still so that the electrocardiograph is not distorted by activity of other muscles, because if they contract it also shows electricity leakage though to the skin. An electrocardiograph is that sensitive it can even pick up the electrical current from the network in the room, which is why modern ECG machines have a device inside that neutralizes this particular hertz of the electricity circuit in the room. With only four electrodes located on your ankles and wrists, you are able to make a simple ECG, but for a more detailed picture you need six extra electrodes. These ones are placed on the chest underneath the heart. Because the electrical impulse changes according to the place where you measure it, every electrode picks up a slightly different signal. By combining the ten signals in 12 different ways you get a realistic image of what is happening inside the heart, which is why we have the name 12 lead ECG.

To take an ECG only takes a couple of minutes and doesn't hurt, although when you have a hairy chest the electrodes pull on them when it is taken off. An electrocardiogram is a graphical display of the way the electrical activity goes through the heart and how it changes during the heart cycle. The heart cycle is the contraction of the atria and immediately after that of the ventricles, and then the relaxation of the heart after it has been contracting. The millimetre squares have a double meaning—in the vertical direction (so from the bottom to the top) you can read in these squares how big or how small the electrical signal is exactly. Two big squares are equal to one millivolt. In the horizontal direction (from left to right) the little squares resemble time, one big square is for 2/10 of a second, which is true if the paper speed is 25mm per second. If you want to see details of every cycle or you want to see bigger then you can change the paper speed and the graphical impulse is spread out over more paper and makes it bigger. If you have a computer, you don't really need to do that, but you are still talking about paper speed. Normally five big squares are one second, but every big square is subdivided into 25 small squares, so that is five rows of five. Vertically one small square is 1/10 of a millivolt. Horizontally one small square is four hundredths of a second. You are reading an ECG from left to right and in that way, you see exactly how the conduction is going over the heart in time.

If you have no clue about an ECG and you look at one, then you see a mountainous picture that repeats itself. First there is a little piece of horizon with a little hill and at the end of that it bends downwards. From that time on the line goes steeply up to a peak, and then as fast as it went up it goes down, a little bit more down than before so it is a little valley. After that you get a horizontal line again with a hill, sometimes there is even a second smaller hill, and after this it all repeats itself. The peak and valleys of a heart cycle are representative of certain processes that happen during a heart cycle and they all have their own name, so we call it a P wave, a QRS complex, the T wave, and sometimes a U wave.

Heart muscle cells contract and relax under the influence of an electrical stimulus that presents itself as a wave over the heart. We call that wave an "action potential". When this travels over the heart the electrical current in and out of a heart cell continuously increases and decreases, and we call that process "depolarization" which means that it increases, and "repolarization" which means that it decreases. Heart muscle cells carry an electrical current. At rest, the inner side of the cell carries a negative current compared to the outer side. If the heart muscle cells are stimulated, they depolarize: the inner side gets positive compared to the outer side, and when that happens the cell will contract and because that happens altogether the whole of the heart is contracting. But you know that there is a little difference in timing between the atria and the ventricles as we discussed before.

With the repolarization process the opposite happens—the heart relaxes and the cells carry a negative current. The first little hill on the ECG is the P wave. That is caused by the depolarization of the atria. The depolarization process is just stalled for a moment when the sinus node activity reaches the AV node, but that takes only four hundredths of a second so you can't see that on the ECG. But as soon as the AV node conducts the impulse to the ventricles, you see on the ECG the so-called QRS complex. This complex is much clearer than the P wave because the ventricles are bigger and carry more muscle and have a more forceful contraction than the atria. The QRS complex shows the depolarization of the ventricles. After the depolarization there is a small moment of electrical rest after which we have the T wave. That is the repolarization of the ventricles, and the repolarization of the atria. They happen at the same time as the QRS complex and therefore not seen on the ECG. Sometimes we still find a small U wave after the T wave but the cause of that is not clear as yet. It is possible that this is a reflection of repolarization of the purkinje fibres. It is not only of interest for the doctor to look how high or how deep the waves are but also to find out how long those processes last. To do this we can have a look at the PR interval which is the time of the start of the P wave to the start of the QRS, and we call it the PR interval (not the PQ interval because the Q wave is often not there). An abnormality in the PR interval can point out an inflammation of the heart muscle whilst a very short PR interval can point out a possible rhythm abnormality like Wolff-Parkinson-White. If the ST segment we discussed in the previous chapter is much higher than normal, you potentially might be suffering an acute heart attack. If it is much lower than normal, then there could be the case of angina pectoris. The QT interval is the contraction of the ventricles and the phase where the heart muscle cells are recuperating. An abnormally long QT interval can be diagnostic for dangerous rhythm.

The exercise ECG

The ECG gives only you an indication of potential problems. Often, we need extra investigations. Angina pectoris and other oxygen related abnormalities can often only be diagnosed when the patient is exercising. That is why we take an ECG during exercise and usually we use a treadmill or a stationary bicycle. The patient is asked to walk or cycle for as long as possible and whilst they do so the resistance of the exercise is increased by the doctor at a certain rate. Usually the test lasts 10 to 20 minutes. The patient is asked to immediately mention if they get complaints, like shortness of breath or chest discomfort or when they are not feeling well. When a stress test is being done there is always a defibrillator and doctor available. A stress test done this way is very safe, but because it is also done in patients where we know they have heart problems, it is much safer if it is done in the right environment. Usually the test is stopped when the patient has reached an amount of exercise that is standard for their age, their body mass index, and their gender, or until they get complaints like chest pains or shortness of breath, and when the electrocardiogram shows abnormalities that are serious. Of course, when you have a young 25-year-old guy, then the level and duration of the exercise are much different than when we talk about exercising an

85-year-old lady. It is however important to go through with the exercise until the moment the person is not able to go any further because then you have the most realistic impression about how the heart is functioning in day to day life. If you stop the exercise too early, it probably does not carry too much value. One thing to realise is that when a stress test like this is normal, then that person probably has no significant heart problems. It is only probable because even when you have a completely normal stress ECG the patient can have a problem down the line because the patient may have atherosclerosis with plaques that do not obstruct the blood flow during the exercise but can still rupture and in that way cause a heart attack.

Holter investigations and other long-term ECG recordings (loop recorders)

An electrocardiogram (ECG) is a representation of the function of the heart at that particular point in time, and sometimes this is too short to see abnormalities. We can deal with this using some techniques to measure the heartbeat over a longer period. In hospital we have that done with a heart monitor but when patients are at home there is wearable registration technology. One of the most used ones is the so-called Holter investigation, named after the American Biophysics Physicist Norman Geoff Holter. You get electrodes on your chest and they are connected to a little device the size of a mobile phone that you can wear day and night at home or at work. During the next 24 to 48 hours the device registers the electrical activity of your heart and puts it on a chip. Usually you are asked to note down your most important activities of your day in a diary. When you go to bed, when you get up, when you do exercise etc. Most Holter recordings also have a little button that you can push which causes a mark on the recording so you can highlight when you felt an extra heartbeat or a palpitation, or chest pains. When the Holter recording is completely normal but you still have complaints, then you can try a so-called event recorder. That is a device like a

Holter that you can wear for weeks and this only has a little button that will activate the recording, but it has a memory that lasts ten minutes or so. Some devices have the ability to send the recording that you made with Bluetooth at the time of the complaints to your doctor. If even the event monitor is not helpful because you only have very sporadic complaints, then the Cardiologist can place a so-called loop recorder. This is a little "USB stick" that he will place under your skin after a local anaesthetic. This little heart rhythm monitor has a battery span of more than three years and can be activated by the patient from the outside with a patient activator when they feel their complaints. It also has a memory lap which means that the recorder has a continuous loop recording of 10 minutes to 30 minutes so that if the patient gets a syncope or faint, the electrical activity during that syncope would still be stored when they regain consciousness. When the loop recorder is not necessary anymore, the Cardiologist can remove it also under a local anaesthetic.

Echocardiogram

With an echocardiogram you can make live images of the heart very easily, and fast, without hurting anybody or any risk to the patient. They use high frequency sound waves, the same as making an ultrasound of a baby in the womb. For the last tens of years the echocardiogram has been one of the most important and most used investigations of the heart because the procedure is relatively cheap, non-invasive, a mobile device—even a handheld device in some instances, and that is a very big difference when you compare it, for instance, to a CT scanner or a PET scanner or MRI. An echo ultrasound teaches you a lot about the structure and the dimensions of the heart, how it is pumping, how the valves are working, and the blood stream. You can see blood clots in the heart, or you can see whether there is fluid in the pericardium or in the lungs. This is one of the best ways to check for congenital abnormalities, problems with the pump, rhythm problems, valve problems, or high blood pressure investigations.

The cone-like sound wave that is produced by bats to localize insects through echolocation is also the same technique used on a medical echo. The difference is that the echo in humans puts the return soundwaves into images. Every tone has another grade in colour in your computer and we call it ultrasound because we use ultrahigh tones that people cannot hear. To make an echocardiogram the investigator asks the patient to take off their shirt and lay down on the bed on their left side. For optimal contact they also put a little bit of gel on the skin and the transducer sensor is then put on the chest looking at the heart. The investigator moves the sensor over the middle of the chest until they find the position that shows the heart very well. Black areas do not produce an echo.

One of the parameters that the specialist can calculate from the echocardiogram is the so-called ejection fraction, the amount of blood that the left ventricle can pump away in one heartbeat. Normally the left ventricle can pump out at least 60% of the maximum amount of blood during each contraction. The doctor can also check the right side of the heart and the rest of the anatomy of the heart. Abnormal structures in one of the four heart cavities can indicate a blood clot. By using the so-called doppler affect, (and you know what that is because if you listen to the changing sound of a siren of an ambulance when they come towards you and when they are going away from you, the difference is the Doppler signal), you can assess which side the blood stream is going, and you can find turbulence around abnormal heart valves. It can also see how thick the heart muscle is and because you can compare an echocardiogram made at rest with an exercise echocardiogram, you can find clues whether the heart gets enough oxygen and hence whether there is a narrowing in the coronary arteries. The exercise echocardiogram can also be done with medication that has a similar effect on the heart as physical exercise. The actual narrowing's are not visible on the echocardiogram.

Another drawback of the echocardiogram is that although the images are very good, they are not as clear as those of a CT or MRI scan, and on top of that, the image is two dimensional—it has no depth. You see only one little slice of the heart each time. But just like 3D pregnancy echo's, a 3D heart echo can give a more complete image. The use of 3D echo, or sometimes even called 4D echo because it also takes into account that the images move therefore adding a time dimension. However, these are used in only a few hospitals at present but is a technique that will evolve and be commonplace. In the old days, the echocardiogram was recorded on a video but is now digital. The technique's evolution is staggering!

Transoesophageal Echocardiography

Instead of having the echocardiographic sender and receiver at the outside of your chest in the transducer, a miniature version can also be put in your chest cavity by means of your oesophagus. It is a similar type of investigation as looking with a camera for ulcers in the stomach. By using the little camera to look at the heart you can see through the back side of the heart and this can be very helpful for people with a lot of fat or lung problems, but also just to have a better look at the structures in the heart that are further away from the chest wall. The ultrasound has only 10 to 15cm penetration into tissues so swallowing a little camera means that the structures of the heart are much clearer because it is the 10 to 15 cm from the back and you don't have to go through the tissue of the chest wall. When you have a transoesophageal echo the doctor usually gives you a little anaesthetic in the back of your throat, so you don't have a problem with your gag reflex.

Duplex investigations

The doctor can also make an ultrasound of the arteries in your neck or your carotid arteries. This is called a duplex investigation because the echogram of the blood vessels are being combined with a measurement of the speed of the blood going through the blood vessels, just as the doppler effect is measuring the speed of the blood-stream inside your heart. The doctor is looking at the possibility of narrowing's in the carotid arteries. If the wall of the artery is too thick or the blood does not go through in the right fashion, then you possibly have atherosclerosis and you have an enhanced risk of having a stroke.

Ankle-arm index

Just by measuring the ankle-arm index, you can determine whether somebody has peripheral vascular disease where there is a narrowing in the blood vessels in t legs. With an ankle-arm index the systolic blood pressure is not only being measured on the upper side of the arms but also at your ankles, and the difference between the two is called the ankle-arm index. Normally the blood pressure in the ankle should be approximately the same as in the arm, but when you have a narrowing in the leg, the blood pressure in the ankle is lower. It takes a little while to do this test because your body has to be at rest when it is happening and before they can do the test, you have to lay for a couple of minutes flat on your back. They put the tourniquets on your arm and on your legs and put a little bit of gel onto your foot. They then listen with a little doppler device to the heartbeat which is detectable in the blood vessels in your feet. The tourniquet on your ankle is then pumped up until the doppler signal, i.e. the heartbeat, has stopped. The tourniquet is emptied and at the moment the doppler signal detects the heartbeat again, it measures the systolic pressure. After this, the same procedure takes place in the arm. The ankle pressure is divided by the arm pressure. If the ankle-arm index is lower than 1 you possibly have a narrowing in your leg artery. They usually perform the measurement a couple of times and take the average.

X-Rays

The x-ray is named after a Dutch-German Physicist called Wilhelm Conrad Röntgen who received the Nobel Prize for physics in 1901 because he found the x-ray that took his name. Röntgen rays have a shorter length than light which we can see and is very easily penetrated in tissues. Dense tissues like bones absorb the Röntgen rays but also a compact muscle like the heart or fluid is visible on an x-ray. What you see on an x-ray are really the reverse shadows of the rays that are being projected on a sensitive medium. Normally those shadows are dark, but x-ray shadows are white or grey. Bones are radiopaque, they absorb the rays, or the rays don't penetrate it, and therefore they produce a very prominent white shadow on the x-ray plate. Air, like in the lungs, is radiolucent so that means it lets a lot of rays pass through which show up as a black shadow. Other materials in the body like blood or fat or muscle tissue and organs are more-or-less grey. An x-ray of the thorax is of the chest where you can see the heart and the lungs, and that is one of the ways the doctor can get an idea about the way the heart looks and the size of it, and possibly of fluid in the lungs.

Usually they make two x-rays, one in the frontal direction of the whole chest and one from the side. The heart is the white/grey spot that is in contrast with the black of the lungs and is usually not wider than 50% of the whole of the chest. If it is wider, that is one of the signs that the heart is enlarged, possibly because the heart is failing or because of a disease of the heart muscle. Also, fluid in the lungs looks like a white/grey spot and that can also be due to a heart abnormality. The coronary arteries can sometimes be seen because there is calcium in the blood vessels and that is absorbed by the x-ray like your ribs and other bones do. In comparison to a CT scan the images of an x-ray are a lot less precise, but the advantage of an x-ray is that you can do it very fast and it is a mobile device that can also be used at the bedside.

CT scan

Compared to an x-ray, a CT scan is a lot more suitable to detect an abnormality of your arteries like an aneurysm. Cardiologists and cardiovascular specialists use this imaging technique, especially to look at the blood vessels of the neck, the head, the heart, and the lungs, but also to look at anatomical abnormalities inside the heart. A CT scanner which is the name of the device (Computer Tomogram scanner), scans the body. It can be compared to a normal x-ray as the cutting machine they use at the bakery to cut your bread versus the bread knife you have at home. The letter C and T of the CT scanner are short for "computer tomography". Tomas is Greek for little plaque and a CT scan is cutting your heart with x-rays in virtual little plaques that can be looked at separately or can be put together to a spectacular 3D image. You don't only need an x-ray source for this but also a big computer. Years ago, CT images were pretty vague, especially if you were looking at moving images like the heart and lungs, but in the present generations there are many more detectors and the computer power has increased tremendously. Still, with all these advantages the best pictures are when you look at the heart during the moment of the diastole when the heart is resting and not contracting. When you make an investigation of your coronary arteries, you are also injected with a contrast medium that contains iodine.

During the scan you lie down on a table that is moved through a small tunnel like a gigantic donut. After the investigation, you can come home immediately or back to your room if you are in hospital. It does not hurt, goes fast, and the images are usually excellent and less prone to artefacts caused by movement than an MRI scan. When you compare an echocardiogram with a CT scan, you cannot only see soft structures but all kinds of structures with a better quality. Disadvantages are the price of a scanner, the fact that the scanner is not mobile, and the increased amount of x-ray that is usually required to make a decent picture. The latter however with modern technology is getting less and less and the amount of x-ray used on the CT scanner is getting very close to a couple of chest x-rays. If you have a CT scan once in a while, that is fine unless you talk about pregnant women, so it is always important to let the x-ray facility know if you are pregnant!

MRI

MRI is short for magnetic resonance imaging. This imaging technique works with electromagnetism and not with x-rays. That is also the big difference with a CT scanner. An MRI scan is less harmful for people that must have a scan very often and it gives similar quality or sometimes even better images. The choice whether you are going to have an MRI or CT scan depends on what the doctor really wants to know. A CT scan is often better to look for abnormalities in the bone, lungs, and chest or to look for cancers. An MRI scan is better in imaging ligaments, problems with the spine or brain tumours, and all in all MRI in principle might be better than a CT scan. However, the technology is a lot more expensive than a CT, it takes more time to do, and because you talk about magnetic fields, the patient cannot have any metals in the body or on the body, so no glasses, no piercings, sometimes a pacemaker can be present but that depends on the type of pacemaker, and it has to be turned to a certain mode during and after the test. An MRI scan of the heart takes at least 30 to 60 minutes and another negative is that during the scan you hear a lot of noise and rattling, although in most centres you do get a headphone to dampen the noise. A variant of the MRI is the MRA which is short for magnetic resonance angiography, and this is a specific investigation to look at the aorta, the coronary arteries, and other big blood vessels in the chest.

Radioisotopes

This investigation works with little radioactive elements, the so-called isotopes. You can localize narrowing's in coronary arteries and damage done after a heart attack and study them, but you can also look for the ejection fraction. The isotopes are infused through your blood stream by putting a little needle in your arm and then injecting the isotopes. They go through the blood and travel through the whole of the body including the heart. Because active myocardial muscle cells need more oxygen and energy than the cells that are less active, they take more radioactive particles and therefore are visualized as coloured dots on the image. There are different forms of isotope investigations with different usages. With a SPECT scan or myocardial scintigraphy, a camera rotates around the patient catching the rays of the patient and transforming it into an image on the computer. In this way, the doctor will get a better idea about the activity and the perfusion of the heart if he is not sure after an exercise investigation and doesn't want to do a cardiac catheterization straight away. The investigation is in two phases, one is done at rest and one after exercise or "medical exercise". During this phase you can see which parts of the heart are not well perfused during the exercise, hence indicating a problem with the blood supply. A PET scan (positron emission tomogram) is not only showing the passing of the blood through the tissue, but also the metabolism and the functioning of the heart as a pump in more detail than a SPECT scan. In this way, a PET scan can show scar tissue after a myocardial infarction. This type of isotope investigation is not dangerous. The radioactive rays are weak and disappear quickly, but because there is not much known about the risk of a foetus, pregnant women usually get a different type of investigation.

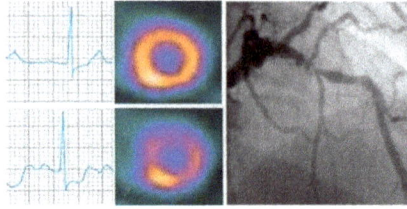

5. This illustration shows 2 ECGs in the left panel. The top one shows the heart with normal blood flow at rest. The bottom one shows abnormalities which represent lack of flow during exercise. The middle panel is the corresponding nuclear image of a cross section of the heart during the nuclear stress test. In the top panel the orange donut suggests a normal perfusion (blood flow); in the bottom panel, the top area has more blue shading, representing lack of blood flow. The right panel is the coronary angiogram where there is a significant narrowing (stenosis) causing no problem when the patient is at rest, but is causing the patient anginal complaints during exercise.

Cardiac catheterization (coronary angiography, coronary biopsies)

A cardiac catheterization is any technique whereby a catheter is used for an investigation or treatment, for instance, percutaneous transluminal angioplasty or for an ablation. The term is also used as synonym for coronary angiography, the best investigation to look into a coronary artery. It is one of the best ways to figure out whether angina pectoris is indeed caused by a problem of the coronary artery. To make the coronary artery visible, the Cardiologist injects some contrast material through the catheter. This contrast material is then visualized by using x-rays. During the procedures I discussed in the last chapter about the use of the balloon and stents, the patient is conscious and can look at the images themselves. You don't see blood vessels, but you see the blood with the contrast material and sometimes the narrowing's that are obstructing the blood flow. Not only can the Cardiologist see the narrowing's, but he can also measure the blood pressure and the oxygen levels in specific heart chambers, he can look for rhythm abnormalities by doing an electrical test, and he can see whether there are little holes on the heart and so forth.

Because there is a risk of damaging the artery, a coronary angiography is only used in people with severe complaints where we cannot look for the cause of the problem in a simpler way. And when you know there is a problem, it is the only way to actually proceed with putting in a balloon or a stent. The investigation usually takes about an hour. Sometimes the doctor takes a little piece of the heart muscle during this test and this biopsy is done with a catheter that has a little beak on the end that can snip a little piece of the heart muscle which is then taken to the lab for further investigation. This is used especially when a heart muscle disease is suspected or in the case of a cardiac transplant to check whether the heart muscle has signs of rejection.

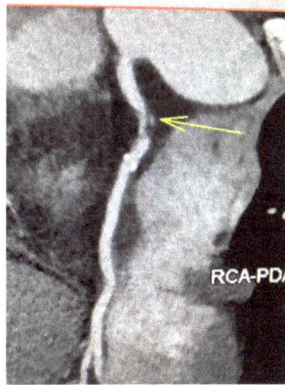

6. This is a CT image (angiogram) of a right coronary artery (RCA) showing a complicated lesion with narrowing of the blood vessel (arrow). This image shows a much better view of the anatomy of plaque compared to an invasive angiogram and this is the reason why a CT coronary angiogram has become very popular since 2015.

Electrophysiological investigations

An electrophysiological investigation (or EP study) is one of the techniques to investigate heart rhythm problems, especially when a normal ECG is not sufficient. They can also be used to investigate the possibility of certain treatments like an ablation, the effect of medication, or what to do with a certain pacemaker tuning. The technique of the EP study is approximately the same as when you have a PTCA. An EP study is done by a specialist and is not done by all Cardiologists. It is done with catheters that are connected to electrodes and brought into the heart by the Cardiologist through a blood vessel, usually from your groin. On the other side the catheters are connected to a computer. In this way the doctor can not only register the heart rhythm, but he can also stimulate the heart to simulate an abnormality or find out where a particular problem in the electricity system is located. It all sounds weird, but the procedure is very controlled and safe in experienced hands. The procedure takes place like the coronary angiogram in the Cardiac Catheterization Laboratory and usually two to four catheters are placed. There is enough space in your blood vessels to take those catheters because they are only a couple of millimetres wide whilst your blood vessels are at least as thick as your pinkie and are even bigger closer to the heart. The Cardiologist usually puts the little electrodes close to the sinus node, the AV node in the right atrium, the coronary sinus which is a big artery between the left atrium and the left ventricle, and the right ventricle. If a rhythm abnormality can be provoked, then the area where it starts and how it travels over the heart can be studied in a very detailed fashion and the Cardiologist can then map the electricity going over the heart. The way it goes differs from person to person. In the meantime, the electrical activity is also measured on the skin on the outside like with an ECG but very fast with a paper speed of 100mm instead of 25mm which is also much more sensitive.

The Cardiologist can tell you the results immediately after the test and whether the abnormalities are amenable for an ablation or whether it needs to be treated in a different way. Sometimes an ablation is immediately done during the EP study. If it is more complicated, then you will have to come back for a new appointment.

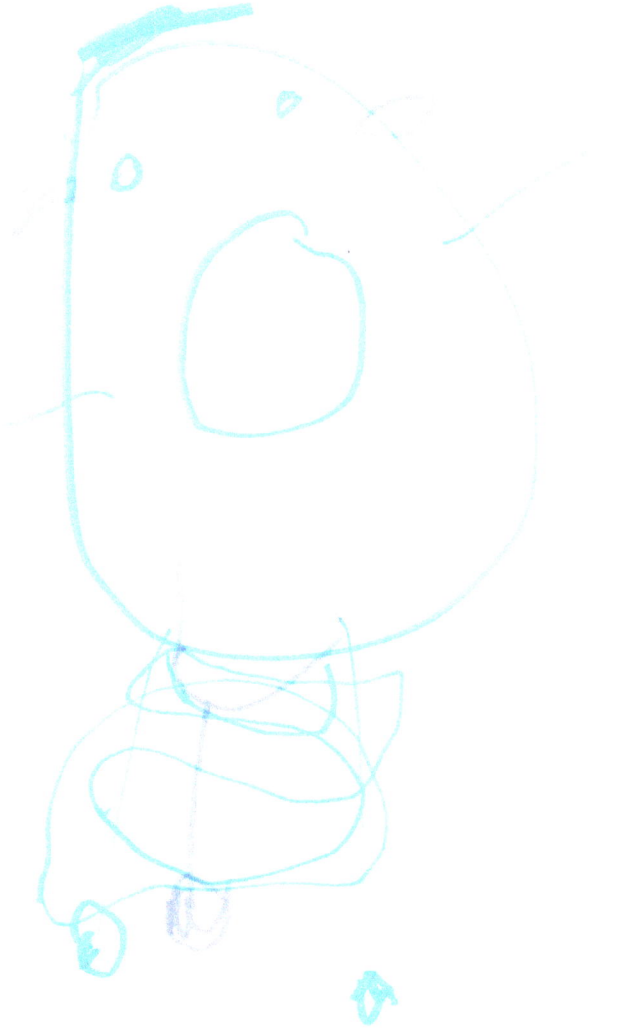

7. Heart doctor by Ayla May

19 PREVENTION OF HEART AND VASCULAR DISEASE—YOU CAN DO A LOT YOURSELF

Primary and secondary prevention

So you now know in principle how your heart and your vessels work in normal circumstances, what the alarm signals are if something in the system is not going accordingly, which kind of investigations they have to do in order to find out construction problems and abnormalities, and how doctors can do things to try and fix electrical and mechanical malfunction, or blood perfusion plumbing problems. We did see that an arrhythmia, a bad working heart valve or a blocked-up artery can occur in isolation but also that they can often influence each other. A malfunction in one technical department of the heart can cause problems in the other two. And then, the most important bit still has to be addressed! Until now we have been talking about the role of the doctor and the Cardiologist but they usually occur on the scene when there is something wrong with the engine of your body, and the question is what can people do themselves and what should they not do, to prevent cardiovascular problems? Which check-ups can you do on your own accord before you have symptoms? Which lifestyle habits should you embrace to prevent heart and blood vessel problems or to help to alleviate them? And which first aid techniques people can offer victims of severe disease after they call the ambulance? So this chapter is about the responsibility of each of us to manage our own heart as well as that of others. Your gender, your race, your age, or genetic predisposition, is something we cannot influence, but you can take it into account and anticipate the risks which are associated with them. All other risk factors are something that are in your domain and you can influence them. Prevention does not only mean to prevent illness, which is so-called primary prevention. You also have secondary prevention; to recognize alarm signals or find problems very early in the piece so you can nip them in the bud and you can undertake action to lower the risk of worsening the problem or make the risk to die from it as little as possible.

Marathons can do, but just sitting less is not too bad either

Regular physical exercise lowers your blood pressure, your choles-terol levels, your weight, and therefore also your risk to have type 2 diabetes and heart and blood vessel problems. Above that, it improves your level of energy, your humour, your resistance, your strength, and your feeling of fitness. That is actually quite a bit. Moving your body around is nothing more and nothing less than an effective and safe way to prevent heart and blood vessel disease, and even to treat them. In 2013 researchers from Harvard University and Stanford Univer-sity looked at more than 300 clinical science projects and they concluded that there is no statistical difference between the positive influences of physical exercise on heart disease compared to the use of medication. Of course, when you are a cardiac patient you should ask your doctor about which type of therapeutic exercise you can do. Another more recent insight in this matter is that you don't have to go to the gym every week for hours on end to punish yourself with exer-cise to get an important effect on your cardiovascular health. In general, the principle that you have to move your body every day for at least 30 minutes in a reasonably intense way to stay healthy is true, but for many people not really practical and definitely not for seven days a week. I think that such advice is sometimes counterproductive because people lose their mojo, or they don't even start to do it. It is much better to have any form of exercise, even a little. Moving around does not cost that much time. An exercise session of ten minutes three times a week with only one minute of very intense movement every time has already shown to have clear health benefits. That is shown in a recent Canadian investigation. In this study two groups of men with a sedentary lifestyle were tested. The first group did a workout of ten minutes three times a week for 12 weeks, two minutes cycling as a warmup, three fast runs on the bicycle of 20 seconds with two minutes easy cycling in between, and after the third sprint to have a cool down on the bicycle for three minutes. The other group of men went three times a week for 45 minutes on a cycling trip reaching 70% of their maximal heart rate. They also had two minutes of warm up and three minutes of cooling down, and they were busy for 50 minutes per training session. In both groups the maximum oxygen uptake was improved, the sensitivity for insulin and the mitochondrial amount in the muscle cells improved as well.

These factors are thought to be important in the relationship with cardiac health, but surprisingly the amount of improvement was the same in both groups. In other words, 30 minutes of interval training per week can have the same effect as training five times as long, so you cannot use lack of time as a reason not to do exercise to improve your overall health. Really if you get down to the nitty gritty, moving is not even a must. If you just stand up instead of sitting down that is already a benefit according to a research program done at the University of Oxford. If you stand every day two hours longer you are lowering your blood sugar levels and your cholesterol levels in your blood considerably. In the western world we sit much too long at home and at work. On average more than half the time that we are awake, we sit. If you sit more than four hours per working day and more than six hours in total it is unhealthy, even if you go to the gym after work. Sitting longer than one hour in one particular position is even unhealthier. It is not only a disaster for your back, but it also brings your body into a kind of shut down mode. Your blood sugar level rises, you are not burning any fat, your blood and your lymph fluids slow down and that increases your risk of getting diabetes, obesitas, and cardiovascular disease. The American investigator James Levine is correct when he says that sitting is the new smoking. You can see that more and more companies are creative in this field with low-high desks, bicycle chairs, walking meetings, and other anti-sit measures or alternatives for traditional office furniture. I think that is a great effort. You should try and make good practice and stand up a couple of times every hour and walk around a bit. That is a very simple, achievable, and free measure. You can make a phone call to lose no time. Also, drink a little bit of water every time because not only it is good for your gut, but you have to get up more often to go to the toilet and gets you out of your chair this way.

Those who want to sit less and find that short intensive workouts are too much, can walk as often as possible during the week to go for half an hour to an hour walk, preferably with a dog. You don't have to go into fancy gym clothes, you don't have to take a shower after you've done it, and it doesn't require special equipment or preparation. It is important to move regularly. Short and intensive or something a little bit longer and more easy-going. It doesn't make a difference as long as you find a way to move that is workable for you. If during your exercise your heartbeat goes up for a while, then that is another plus. If you walk at the speed of 5km an hour, then you definitely will also increase your heart rate.

Physical exercise can mean doing a sport, but that is not necessarily the case. Playing a sport does not give you much extra profit just for your physical wellness in comparison to other more mundane or non-competitive forms of moving that we usually do not call a sport. This includes activities like walking, cycling, swimming, making love, or working in the garden. Also work where you are not sitting in front of the computer all day long at a desk, behind a car steering wheel or other machinery is counted as physical exercise. By the way, sport can also entail medical risks if you use bad equipment or without the right advice or start to continuously increase the levels. The Dutch biologist Midas Dekkers has had a crusade for many years against the "homo athlete" because he noticed in the animal world that animals that do not do "sport" are doing very well as far as longevity. Mr Dekkers is right that sport is in essence not natural, but he does forget that our whole lifestyle is not natural and that most animals in the wild have to move much more than we do, even though it is just to get food or not being eaten themselves. Those animals get enough "sport" in any case. Sport has definite benefits that other forms of exercise do not have. Sport is usually more exciting and more challenging than going for a walk because of the competition element. For instance, if you play tennis, the chance is there that you want to see a top match on television and that increases your pleasure to try and improve your technique, taking lessons, or going to the tennis court more often, so slowly you are going to be part of a tennis culture. You are a member of a club of tennis players and the same is true for people that have cycling as a sport or people that run marathons. If you play sport in a group or with a partner you also have positive pressure to really start on the day and time that you said you would, even though it might be raining or you are not feeling like it that day. Also, through sport you can make new friends and have a rich and fulfilling social life. That altogether brings you in an upward spiral.

But I have to say, do whatever you like most. That will mean that you are going to continue it for longer. Maybe it is a sport or an activity that you did in your earlier life but have given up because of work commitments or maybe it is something that you always wanted to try like fencing? Choose a form of exercise that you can do at home or close in the neighbourhood for the whole year and maybe at different times of the day or the week. This will mean that the resistance to start the activity or to continue the activity is as low as possible. As with many things in life, variation is the key to continue to like something, so regularly try new activities, move with your favourite music or in company you enjoy. Don't spend your money on very expensive sport gadgets or magazines but do invest in decent equipment—a pair of comfortable walking or running shoes for instance. It is you who makes the choice. My own preference is a combination of activities, I play tennis, play golf with the kids, and go for daily walks with the dog. His name is Olaf.

How intensely should a human being exercise?

The practical rule of thumb is that the intensity of the exercise is okay if it is low enough to continue having a conversation but too high to be able to sing. Whatever it is that you do, always start with a short warmup and end with a couple of minutes cool down, so don't go and sit down straight away, stand still or lay down after a decent exercise, otherwise you can get dizzy or get palpitations or get painful muscles. Just use your little grey cells. If you are middle aged and you have too many kilos and you didn't exercise for years on end and you are fed up of pulling your belly in in front of the mirror, then it is not very smart to, in a euphoria of mind, suddenly, three to four times a week to go for a jog until your tongue is on our shoes, even when you start slowly. For sure, you are jogging your knees all the way to the Orthopaedic Surgeon. Because you really have to exercise a lot to lose any amount of weight, it can also come with extra frustration, because after that you sit again with a meniscus or other knee problem and still have all the fat rolls on top of your belt. This kind of scenario is the shortest way to a new period of complete inactivity! If you didn't do physical exercise for a while and you are too heavy, then you have to really start very slowly with short walks for instance or 15 minutes on the home trainer or just a couple of laps in the swimming pool. You have to give your body the time to get used to that new, more energetic boss. Your body spent years to go from a fit teenager to a couch potato. You can't reverse that straight away. It is a matter of months, and as you get fitter you can slowly increase the amount of stress you put on your heart muscles and joints, and if you are already feeling some problems in your joints (most people 40 or older have cartilage problems) then in that case swimming, walking, or cycling is a good idea as a start. During a later phase you can think about maybe intensifying your walking, going for a run, or other activities whereby you are putting more pressure on your bones. Putting pressure on your bones is a good way to also make your skeleton healthier and that reverses the risk of osteoporosis. Slender women can especially find a lot of benefit from that.

I have one last piece of advice for people who want to go into sports or are already in sports: go and see a sport physician and get advice on a more active life whatever your goal might be. One is going to run a marathon, the other is going to have a cycle around the local park. The Australian Institute of Sports and your GP would be a good starting point to also check what your risks are for sport and what your best sport would be for your heart health and your general physique. There are some websites as well that will answer questions regarding starting a sport and that might be a good start to prevent disillusionment.

20 NON-SMOKERS ARE LOOKING MUCH SEXIER AND THEY ARE BETTER BETWEEN THE SHEETS!

S hall I state the obvious? Don't smoke. Don't start, or stop it now if you want to prevent developing a heart or blood vessel problem. The chemical substances in tobacco smoke damage the inner lining of your blood vessels and what happens is that very early in the piece they calcify and collect more rubbish. Because the CO_2 is taking the place of the oxygen, your heart is unnecessarily put under a heavy load. Apart from that, your blood clogs up faster if you smoke, and that means you have more risk of having a heart attack or a stroke.

The more you smoke the greater the problem, but less smoking does not keep you out of the danger zone. Passive smoking is also detrimental and even in a room or car where there has been smoking earlier is detrimental. There is also something not like second-hand, but third-hand smoke that consists of remnants of nicotine and other chemical stuff present in tobacco smoke. This mingles with the dust in your house and other "normal" dirt in the interior of places where someone smoked, like your carpets, your curtains, car seats, but also smooth surfaces like the kitchen bench and the table. Research has shown that in this "old smoke" all kinds of cancer promoting chemicals are found which are a real risk, especially for kids. It does not help to get fresh air in rooms where smoking took place, the smell might go but the dangerous chemicals are still there. It takes weeks with very intense cleaning and a lot of money associated with that, to try and clean the house where smoking occurred. There is only one good way to prevent third-hand smoke and that is to never smoke inside. But the facts are what they are.

Approximately one in five deaths by heart and vascular disease is the direct effect of smoking. Smokers have two to four times the risk of getting cerebral vascular disease, and twice the risk to have a heart attack or a stroke. In women who smoke and use oral anticonception that danger is even larger. And we haven't even touched on all the different forms of cancer and lung disease that are caused by smoking or being aggravated by smoke. Smoking can damage any organ and every cell in your body. Do you get the picture? I am not talking much more about this and I presume that stopping smoking for the most addicted smokers is not a matter of they don't want to smoke or know that smoking is bad, but that the addiction is that bad that they can't. Therefore, it is probably not that smart to try to prevent smoking or to scare smokers by putting horrible pictures on the cigarette packages. I think that people are getting used to those pictures and that they are less and less useful in the end. I think that campaigns against smoking should focus on all the advantages of not smoking for your inner health, but also for your outer health—your fresh breath and your sex life.

Smoking makes people grey and it ages the skin. Smokers are on average one-and-a-half years older than non-smokers of the same age. Smoking increases your risk to psoriasis by 20%, it makes your teeth and fingers yellow and your hair thinner. Smokers get grey earlier and, last but not least, smoking induces impotence, but also bacterial vaginal infections and it reduces the libido of both genders considerably.

In short, the message is that non-smokers are looking on average a lot sexier and are more easily kissed because of their fresh breath, and they will do much better in bed! But stopping smoking for many people is extremely difficult and that is not rocket science. The nicotine in the smoke increases the level of dopamine in your brain which is a nerve transmitter that plays an important role in the feel good mechanism, and it is therefore also part of the mechanism of people who are hooked on cocaine or heroin. Smokers who want to stop smoking not only have to kick this nicotine rush, but also the whole ritual that is associated with smoking, the buying of the tobacco— often at specific places in combination with other fun things like candy, booze, or your favourite magazine, the opening of a new smelling package of cigarettes or tobacco, the getting hold of the cigarette in the packet and putting it between your lips, the magic of fire of the cool Zippo, the little sound of the tobacco being burned, the prickling scent, the chewing on the smoke in your mouth, the little ring that you can blow out, manipulate the cigarette or the cigar or the pipe, playing with it, the inhaling, the immediate kick, the ticking of the cigarette to get rid of the ash ... Those who have smoked 20 cigarettes a day for 25 years have done this very refined ritual 182,5000 times and have sucked smoke into their lungs more than 3.6 million times, that habit is really carved into your body. Your body and mind are completely dependent on this ritual and want to keep it this way, and despite all the campaigns and the prohibition of smoking in public buildings, cafes, restaurants, one in five Australians continue to smoke with an average of 16 cigarettes a day!

The good news is that the positive effects of stopping smoking start immediately after your last puff. After 20 minutes your blood pressure is lower, and after eight hours the oxygen uptake in your blood has normalized. A smoker who can stop using that particular cigarette in the morning before exercise will recognize immediately that they have a better exercise capacity that same day. After three days of stopping, your breathing is a lot better and you are less short of breath. After three months your blood flow is really improved, and a year after you stop your risk of a heart attack has lowered by 50%, and after five years you have halved your risk for a stroke. After 15 years your risk to die from the smoking inhalation is no longer higher than somebody who never smoked and, by the same token, you have saved yourself a couple of thousand dollars. Hey isn't that great? How long or how much you have smoked, the advantages of stopping are gigantic for both your body and your wallet. It is never too late to stop.

There are many books, websites, and specialists who can help you stop this expensive, dangerous, smelly, and asocial habit called smoking. I smoked when I was younger, and I stopped from one day to the other day. There are many people who can do it that way. You also have some people who can smoke once in a while. Partly because there is a genetic component that dictates how long the brains of a smoker need nicotine. The longer that effect lasts, the less sooner you want to have a new cigarette. For me personally this once in a while smoking didn't work, but also in general you have to stop completely to deal with the dangerous effects. Don't get sucked into things like making an interim solution like going from cigarettes to rolling tobacco or lower nicotine cigarettes, cigarillos, the water pipe, or cannabis. All these alternatives carry the same danger. There are some people who can use nicotine plasters or e-cigarettes and use that as a step to stop. The well-dosed and slowly diminished amount of nicotine in nicotine-plasters has shown to work and this is also important because some people are really afraid to gain more weight which is for many smokers a reason not to stop. Also, medication can be very useful if stopping smoking is not working any other way. It works in any case to make a plan, to write down why you want to stop and get rid of everything related to smoking in your house . You have to make a date when you are going to stop and you have to share this with family and friends so they can help you with this, and you have to use your Facebook connections to help you with stopping. If you really want to have a cigarette take a deep breath, hold it for ten seconds, and repeat it a couple of times until your desire to smoke is reduced. That does work. It is also useful to have sugar free candies or healthy snacks nearby because you might need to distract from your smoking thoughts and give your hands and your mouth something else to do. You have to realise that it is really going to be difficult and that you will suffer cold turkey effects, irritation, stress, more hunger, concentration problems etc. in the beginning, but these cold turkey symptoms are going to be less and less and within two weeks usually gone. Still, the desire to smoke can come back for years in certain circumstances. Those are the weak moments, the times where you used to smoke in the early days like in the morning with your first nice fresh coffee, the nice cigarette after food, smoking in a traffic jam, or after going to the cinema. Most smokers who stop have to try three times and it is not a disaster if you fail and restart smoking, but you have to try again. Every day without tobacco smoke is a day that your health is advancing. Just start again with your plan and ask yourself what you are going to do next if you feel that you have to smoke again.

Only one to two glasses a day

It's a million-dollar question. Is alcohol used in moderation good or not good for your heart? The best-known positive effect is a slight elevation of your "good cholesterol" the HDL, but also regular exercise can cause an increase in your HDL. It is also said that drinking would prevent thrombosis. It is not clear whether it is only chemicals in red wine like flavonoids and other antioxidants that give cardiovascular protection, or the ethanol itself which is also present in other alcoholic beverages. There are over 100 studies that give positive arguments to drink one or two glasses of alcohol daily. The most recent important study that I saw regarding this subject, indeed confirms that not all but a lot of cardiovascular problems are less frequent in people that use alcohol in a moderate way, comparing people who don't drink at all to people who drink heavily. But we

have to stay honest: there are no well-done large scale scientific investigations that are able to isolate the drinking of wine or alcohol in
general as a separate positive measure to differentiate that from other
factors like healthy lifestyle, healthy food, exercise, and so forth.
They just don't exist. When you look at the risk categories of non-
drinkers there are also a lot of former drinkers which means that the
result of the investigations might not be as clear. It also does not take
into consideration that an increase in alcohol consumption can
increase the risk of breast cancer, even when you use alcohol in
moderation. But one thing is clear, when you drink too much alcohol
—more than two glasses a day for a man and more than one glass a
day for a woman—it is not healthy. A lot of people make the mistake
to think that if they drink 14 glasses of wine or beer in a weekend that
that is okay if they don't consume any alcohol during the other five
days of the week, because they are still only having an average of two
a day. That is not true. When we use moderation, it may have a
particular advantage, especially in people who are 40 plus, but it is
never alright to drink on any given day more than one or two glasses
of alcohol. When you misuse alcohol your lipids in your blood go up,
you get obesitas, you get high blood pressure. In men more than 10%
of cases of high blood pressure is caused by alcohol use. Alcohol is
also considered to be an important cause of a disease of the
myocardium that can cause congestive heart failure and serious
rhythm abnormalities. Chronic alcohol use as well as sudden excess
alcohol (binge drinking) is detrimental to the heart.

Apart from that there is a whole long list of other alcohol related
medical problems and this goes from all kinds of cancer, gout, osteoporosis, a lot of psychological damage, and then we haven't discussed
the social impact, the lack of work, the crisis in your relationship, the
domestic violence, and the child abuse related to alcohol.

Last but not least, all the deadly traffic accidents of which more than
half is related to use of alcohol. So maybe you're interested as the
reader to find out what I do myself? Well, I do like to have a glass of

wine and, at the same time, I advise people not to overdo it, not only in the short but also not in the long term. I advise people younger than 40 who do not drink to keep it that way. The risk of heart and blood vessel disease is however a very complicated maze of all kinds of influences that you do have control over but also a lot of factors that are outside your control. In the ideal world we don't have to deal with genetic predisposition. In the ideal world we don't smoke, we don't drink alcohol, we have a normal body mass index, we do not have diabetes, we eat healthily, and we move and exercise sufficiently. If one of those factors are not being met, then you might want to keep the other parameters maximally under control, and even more so if they are factors that you cannot have influence on like getting older or genetic predisposition. Together with your doctor you will have to discuss those different factors and then discuss what is possible and what is desirable. The result of that should be a double-edged sword —at one side you have to reduce your cardiovascular risk, but also you have to stay a happy human being. In my opinion, the costs of some pleasure are worth risking for a longer and happier life.

A risk profile has to be done per individual. You cannot have general advice that will suit everybody like a glove. I am also just a human being and I give myself the advantage of doubt and I think at my age one or two glasses of red wine or alcohol standard drinks cannot harm me too much and might even have some advantages. In the meantime, I am not smoking, I am eating reasonably healthily, and I exercise regularly. A smoker or drinker that is over 80 who would like to live a couple more years happy without a heart attack or a stroke, would be much better off however to stop eating and drinking unhealthily. But if it costs them that much effort that they are going to be a "frustrated bitch or bastard" then it is altogether probably defendable if they continue these habits, however, they should still walk around the block with their dog and see their GP regularly.

21 LESS IS BETTER THAN MORE AND SWEET IS WORSE THAN FAT

The scientific discussion about the positive effect of moderate alcohol use in the sense of reducing cardiovascular risk is small in comparison to the many different opinions about healthy or not healthy food. About fats as well as carbohydrates and proteins, you find very conflicting opinions of experts in the field. For years we heard that plant-based fats were more ideal over animal fat, and therefore we had to use plant-based margarine instead of butter: today a lot of studies make a plea for the opposite. In the old days you had to avoid fat and you had to count calories to lose weight. Today it is predominantly sugar which is the culprit. One day you read that wheat products are healthy, the other day you read that you have to really steer clear of carbohydrates. Hello? People don't know any more what they have to believe. They lose their trust in science and they turn to promising wonder diets that usually do not work, or because everything is too hard they go back to their old way of living which was the one they wanted to change to start with. Does that mean that all the studies and scientists are barking up the wrong tree? Well obviously a few of them do because their opinions are 100% opposite each other. Butter cannot be healthy and at the same time not healthy. Certain food items of course can have pros and cons. I think that people who preach revolutionary or extreme food ideas have a great responsibility and have to be really careful that they do not cause more confusion than give people more insight and a way forward to better health. What I think is especially bad are those suggestions which are unrealistic as far as our food patterns are concerned, notwithstanding the fact that many of these advices have no scientific grounds, they also need to realise that eating, putting food on the table, is not only a matter of health but also one with an organizational side, a practical side, social, and financial side. You have to have the time to buy the right ingredients, you have to have the time to make a proper meal, you have to take into account the different tastes of the people that you are feeding, you need to have the time to put something different on the table every day to make it interesting, and it has to all fit within your budget. To give advice to people about the feeding patterns that are scientifically just, but in practice impossible to maintain, like eating no bread for instance, also do not cut the mustard.

Before we talk further about my personal tips in what to eat, I would like to discuss briefly how our nutrition actually works. Often studies and articles about nutrition and food are not that clear or are old-fashioned. I would like to spend a few moments on this fascinating subject to highlight a couple of issues which you might have always found interesting but too hard to sort out exactly. Nutrition is not everything in our life, but it is very much of our life. Everything that is alive has to get their hands on energy one way or another. If you don't eat, then you get weak and then you die. The food we eat is varied, but it really is only a couple of basic elements: carbohydrates, proteins, fats, vitamins, minerals, fibres, and water. Some food categories which have been treated in an industrial fashion also contain artificial taste or colour materials and preservatives. But of course, these are not part of our natural nutrition.

Carbohydrates

Let's start with the carbohydrates or saccharides, the basic fuel of our body. Carbohydrates consist of carbon, hydrogen, and oxygen atoms in both simple and complex structures. The simplest form is glucose or dextrose. Glucose is a kind of sugar which can be absorbed in your blood, so it is available for your cells. The cells take in the glucose and convert it into energy. We call glucose a sugar because this glucose tastes sweet.

There are other carbohydrates than sugars, although these two terms are used indiscriminately. Just like glucose, fructose is a simple sugar, a so-called monosaccharide. Fructose, which is the most important sugar in fruit, has the same chemical formula as glucose ($C_6H_{12}O_6$) but the atoms are organized differently in the molecule. A more complex sugar is sucrose or saccharose. Those are the scientific names of the product that we all know as the sugar we use on our table. Sucrose, saccharose, caster sugar, cane sugar, pearl sugar, it is all the same stuff—a combination of glucose and fructose. Lactose you might know from the term "lactose intolerance" which is the inability to digest mild sugar. Lactose is a chemical combination of glucose and galactose. This last one is just like glucose and fructose, a monosaccharide or simple sugar. You also have maltose, a sugar which is made of two glucose atoms together. The monosaccharides glucose, fructose and galactose are the only carbohydrates that can be absorbed in blood through the wall of your gut. Lactose, sucrose and maltose are disaccharides which have to be consumed by enzymes in your digestive tract first into monosaccharides before they can be absorbed in the blood. Mono and disaccharides are both still simple carbohydrates.

So apart from the simple carbohydrates you also have complex carbohydrates, those are long glucose molecules that we call starch, which is the form in which plants lock in their energy. Grains like corn, wheat, or rice, but also potatoes and bananas contain a lot of starch.

Your digestive system in your gut breaks down these complex carbo-hydrates until they end up being glucose molecules. That is why the digestion of starch takes longer. If you drink a sugar-rich soft drink, then that glucose gets into your blood with a speed of some tens of calories per minute. However, when you eat a complex carbohydrate then only a few calories are absorbed in your blood stream per minute. Especially in kids, you see the effect of simple short sugars very well. If kids snack on candy or drink a soft drink, then their blood sugars rise very quickly. The pancreas reacts on that by making a lot of insulin which is why the blood sugars will drop as fast as they were rising. That low sugar level can last for hours and that will cause the adrenalin level to increase which has an effect in kids to make them nervous and itchy and bad-tempered. So, you can see here that what food you eat influences your emotions because it has effects on your hormone levels.

Insulin takes care that glucose gets from the blood into your cells. This hormone also converts glucose into glycogen that can be stored in your liver and your muscles. This helps to convert excess glucose into fat and prevents proteins being broken down to be used as a source of energy. In short, glucose is such an important energy provider that our body has all kinds of regulatory mechanisms to keep blood sugar at the right level in your body.

Carbohydrates are very much under scrutiny these days, to say it politely. Some government suggestions claim that you have to get half of your calories out of carbohydrates. Other specialists argue, however, that it makes you fat and that risks getting type 2 diabetes from carbohydrates. For both opinions you can find pretty good argu-ments—it depends from person to person, but also from carbohydrate to carbohydrate. If you feel that from reading the previous text short or simple carbohydrates are not as healthy as the longer complex carbohydrates, then I need to rephrase that, because short sugars in fruit are less harmful than complex sugars in bread or pasta made of white flour. The difference between the carbohydrates and the refined carbohydrates is much more useful. If you have unrefined carbohydrates, then we talk about the carbohydrates that you find in natural fibre rich non-industrial nutrients like vegetables, fruit, nuts, and grains. Refined carbohydrates you find predominantly in products which have had an industrial treatment like products where they artificially remove natural fibres as in sugar, e.g. soft drinks, fruit drinks, white bread, pastry, white pasta, and white rice. If you eat too much of these you are indeed at risk of obesity and type 2 diabetes, especially if you have a certain affinity to get that easily, and this of course carries all kinds of risk for the development of heart and blood vessel problems. Refined carbohydrates play volleyball with your blood sugar. It affects the way you experience appetite and how much you long for sugar, as I explained in the example of the kids. Apart from this, products with a lot of refined sugars don't usually have many other useful healthy nutrition. If you take complex and non-refined carbohydrates, then you find they are full of nutrients which you can recommend. Why are there then so many diets that advocate a feeding pattern with a few or even no carbohydrates at all, and the person has to eat a lot of proteins and fats?

At least 20 well-performed studies have shown that carbohydrate-poor diets work better for people who are overweight than diets without fat and that they are also better when you look at your HDL cholesterol, your triglycerides, your blood sugar, and your blood pressure. In other words, carbohydrate-poor diets are also better for your heart. People who are overweight and have type 2 diabetes, or another reason to have a higher risk of developing cardiovascular problems, then they can definitely benefit by having a carbohydrate-less feeding pattern. They only have to find a way to maintain that diet. People who do not have cardiovascular problems but they want to keep their cardiovascular health in check, can also benefit by using less carbohydrates but they can permit themselves a little bit more and don't have to worry that much about non-refined or refined carbohydrates. For instance, non-refined sugars do not make you fat or give you diabetes—refined sugars do that. For thousands of years humans have consumed carbohydrates but the obesity and diabetes problem only started some decennia ago, which is not a surprise if you realise that the nutritional industry started to produce a lot of refined "fake food"—the worst are all those very sweet fruit yoghurts with zero percent fat, or vegetarian meatballs with zero percent meat but a lot of refined sugars! We do not really need carbohydrates, in itself it is not an essential nutrient. Our brains can use fatty acids and use ketones as an energy source. The little bit of glucose that our brain needs can be produced by our body itself with a process called gluconeogenesis. But if you would not eat any carbohydrates at all, also no complex ones, then we would have to get many other important nutrients which we do get out of the carbohydrate rich products by alternative routes like fibre and vitamins.

Proteins

We have carbohydrates that support the cells' energy, but proteins give them the construction material they need to grow and maintain their structure. Apart from this, proteins have many other functions. They are building materials, they deconstruct building materials, they change building materials, or they safeguard which items can get into a cell and which items have to leave a cell. Chemically, proteins are chains of essential and not essential amino acids. The latter category your body can make. The essential amino acids you have to ingest through plant or animal nutrition. Meat, milk, eggs provide us with so-called complex proteins because they all contain essential amino acids. You find those less in plant derived foods, but because you can combine different types of plants you can still get to enough of the essential amino acids during the day. Nuts, beans and soy, for instance, contain a lot of different proteins. Your gut will break down these proteins until the amino acids contained within can subsequently be absorbed in your blood stream. How many proteins you need depends on the person, but on average a person of 70kg would need about 50 grams of proteins daily. You will have this with a can of tuna, a glass of milk, and one sandwich, and that would set you up for the day. These are of course, average values—people who are very active will need more proteins, and the same holds true for healthy octogenarians and people who are recuperating from an injury or operation.

Fat

I am sure you have heard about saturated fat and non-saturated fats, or fatty acids—the most important component of fats. These fats have nothing to do with your feeling of satisfaction fullness, but with a chemical structure of fatty acids. A fatty acid is a strain of carbon atoms and when they are maximally bound to hydrogen atoms, we call them saturated, so they are saturated with H atoms. When you talk about non-saturated fats that is not the case. Most animal fatty acids except those of fish mainly contain saturated fats. The fatty acids in fish are just like those in plants, in general non-saturated. You will also note that saturated fats are usually more solid at room temperature, whilst non-saturated fatty acids often stay fluid at 20 degrees Celsius. How is it possible that margarine or baking butter is not fluid? Because these products contain plant-derived fatty acids which predominantly are non-saturated and therefore should be fluid. Margarine is the way it looks because it is partially hydrogenated which is a chemical process whereby a non-saturated binding is transformed into a saturated binding, and during this process there are so-called trans-fatty acids produced which are the worst ones of all types of fats. Hydrogenation is a technique to make firm fatty acids from fluid fatty acids that you can put on your sandwich but can also be kept longer with this process. One margarine is not the same as the other margarine, they are not all bad, but I would be very careful with the usage.

Trans-fatty acids contribute to the development of diabetes and increased amount of abdominal fat and this increases your risk of developing heart and vascular disease considerably. Fatty acids can be simple or complex and saturated. Simple unsaturated fatty acids have one couple of C atoms with a double binding. The complex unsaturated fatty acids have at least two of them. The complex unsaturated fatty acids are divided in omega 3 and omega 6 fatty acids. In our food we often find different types of fatty acids. On the label of the bottle of olive oil in my kitchen, for instance, you will find that it has 18% saturated fats. These are therefore resolved in 82% unsaturated fat. Butter contains 65% saturated and 5% complex unsaturated and 30% simple unsaturated fats but, for whatever reason, the butter is labelled as saturated. If you look at the published effects of these fats on our cardiovascular health you will find again a lot of discussion. Most nutritional specialists find that plant-derived fatty acids are better than animal derived fatty acids and that non-saturated fatty acids are healthier than saturated fatty acids, and that simple unsaturated fatty acids are healthier than complex unsaturated fatty acids, and that omega 3 fatty acids are healthier than omega 6. So, what do you make of all that?

Every fatty acid contains one glycerol molecule and three fatty acids which can be saturated, simple unsaturated, or complex unsaturated. Fats are always combinations of this. Olive oil also contains saturated fat and in cow's meat you also find unsaturated fats. It is a matter of how much of each is present. When during the last century more and more people were suffering heart attacks, investigators looked for a cause and they found that saturated fats increased the cholesterol level in the blood. They knew that cholesterol is a product that was associated with a high risk of the occurrence of heart and blood vessel disease, so they said that saturated fats enhance the risk of the development of cardiovascular disease. Job done. It was a conclusion based on logical thinking, but they were hypothesizing, and it was conveyed in a big way to the public opinion. To find scientific experimental investigations that show without a doubt that consuming saturated fats causes heart and blood vessel disease are not available, not even today, so the exact cause of coronary artery disease is not known as yet. If you eat saturated fat, more recent studies suggest it does not only elevate the so-called bad low-density cholesterol (LDL) but also the "good" (HDL) cholesterol. As I explained previously in this book, there is really in essence only one type of cholesterol and the issue is how this essential substance is packaged to be able to get absorbed in the blood stream. In the old days doctors only measured the total cholesterol level. Later they found that LDL increases the risk of heart and blood vessel disease, but that HDL lowers that same risk. In other words, your total cholesterol level is not saying too much about your cardiovascular risk. In the meantime we have gone a little bit further and we know that LDL is not always bad because there are several sub-types, so you have small LDL and you have large LDL, and it is perhaps only the small LDL which is able to get through the lining of your artery causing damage. People that are predominantly taking in small LDL particles have three times as high risk to have a cardiovascular incident than people with large LDL particles. So does this now mean that we have to throw everything that we learned before about the occurrence of coronary artery disease and the unproven use of fats in the bin? Because most Cardiologists and nutritional experts are hammering into us the perceived correlation between high cholesterol animal fats (apart from fish) and the occurrence of coronary artery disease. They base their opinion on different investigations and in the meantime, we know that a lot of scientific research about health can be muddled by many factors.

The problem with the risk of cardiovascular disease is that a lot of people have a combination of multiple risk factors, they are not only obese but they also eat the wrong food, the wrong fats, they don't move enough, they have a genetic predisposition (family history) etc. It is very hard to isolate only a single factor and keep all other variables constant, and then look which influence of that particular factor is on the cardiovascular risk. And then you have to look for all these items in enough people who you need to contrast with people who do not have the problem over a period which is long enough in time. So people with a genetic abnormality like familial hypercholestero-laemia would do well to watch their cholesterol very strictly, even though we should revisit our opinion about saturated fats. We know for sure that they are better able to withstand heat and that is a reason why they may be much better for broiling and baking.

With the complex non-saturated fats, the relation between omega 3 and omega 6 fatty acids is of importance. Although we do need both fatty acids because they are essential fatty acids, we usually have between 15 to 20 times too much omega 6 by means of certain oils like soy, sunflower, and corn oil. We get that because we use it in the kitchen, but more importantly, through industrially made nutritional products like chips and dressings for the salad etc. On top of that we eat far too much meat of animals who are bulk fed with a lot of omega 6. This imbalance between the omega 3 and omega 6 increases the risk of development of heart and blood vessel disease, cancer, infec-tion, and autoimmune disease. I will not go into detail in the complex chemical process, but omega 6 does not necessarily have to be unhealthy as long as we have enough omega 3. A ratio of 1:1 would be ideal. The best way I feel to make sure that you keep the balance in check is to regularly eat fatty fish, olive or coconut oil instead of other oils, and eat as little industrial made food as possible. This would also be a great tactic to reduce the amount of trans-fatty acids that you might consume.

Fats and fatty acids are a very powerful source of energy. They give us double the number of calories per gram compared to carbohy-drates or proteins. You do need fats as fuel but also because some vitamins which are soluble in fat only get into our body if we consume the fat, and the same is true for some essential amino acids.

Vitamins and minerals

Vitamins are really micronutrients in comparison to macronutrients like fats, proteins, and carbohydrates. We call them that because vitamins are not needed in big quantities, but they are essential. We cannot live without them. Vitamins are no source of energy and are not used as building blocks in our body, but they contribute to the growth, the recuperation and the functioning of our body and our cells. we can make vitamin D ourselves if we get into the sun enough, but most other vitamins we have to get out of our food. We really need at least 13 vitamins. We need A and B which has eight separate fractions, C, D, E and K. If we have not enough of a vitamin, it can cause all kinds of problems, for example, night blindness, skin problems, anaemia, scurvy, or problems with anticoagulation and coagulation (bleeding disorders).

The second type of micronutrients that we need to get out of our nutrition and food are the minerals. The minerals are used by our body to make molecules that we cannot miss. Some very important minerals are calcium, copper, iron, magnesium, phosphate, potassium, selenium, sodium, and zinc. Calcium is not to be missed for the build-up and maintenance of our skeleton, but it also plays an important role in the electricity from the heart just like sodium and potassium.

Fibre

The second last basic element of our nutrition is fibre which we cannot digest but still need. The most important fibres in our nutrition are cellulose, hemicellulose, and pectin. Hemicellulose is present in the coating of diverse amounts of grains like wheat. Cellulose is the complex carbohydrate that gives plants their structure. Pectin you find in fruits especially.

The most important function of fibres in our body is the function that you find least mentioned in texts about healthy nutrition; they are essential for a healthy gut microbiome. It may sound weird, but a human body consists only for a tiny bit out of 'human material'. Your body has many more bacteria than cells—approximately ten times more than human cells. Those bacteria are on your skin, in your mouth, in your nose, but also in your gut. You have more than 500 different types of bacteria in your gut and together we call that the gut "microbiome". Your body gives shelter to ten billion bacteria and they will therefore do all kinds of tasks, like keep your body weight stable, your blood sugar level stable, improve your immunity, and even your brain function. The problem is of course that just like all other forms of life, bacteria need energy, but by the time our food gets into our colon, most of the carbohydrates, proteins, and fats are already taken in our blood stream and there is not enough of these items to supply your microbiome with food, except for fibres. We cannot digest them, but our gut bacteria can. So the fibres in our food are there to feed the non-human part of your body and through your good bacteria have a whole list of positive effects. They feed the cells of your colon and they reduce the inflammation processes in case you have an irritable bowel syndrome or the illness of Crohn or colitis ulcerosa.

Another positive effect of the fibres is that they give you a feeling of fullness and that means that you will take less calorie intake. Nutrition that is rich in fibre has also a lower glycemic index which means that these fibres reduce the amount of peaks in your blood sugar level after a meal with a lot of carbohydrates. Fibres can also lower your cholesterol levels, although the effect on your cholesterol is not as high as was presumed in the old days. There are several studies showing that if you have a diet with a lot of fibre, your risk of development of heart and blood vessel disease is lower. A drawback of this is that bacteria which ferment fibres also produce gas. You will fart more and sometimes you get some pain in your tummy, but that will go away. The common knowledge that fibres will improve your toilet habits and help against constipation and diarrhea is definitely not proven. Also, significant protection against occurrence of colon carcinoma has not been proven. But in any case, having nutrition with a lot of fibre is healthier than nutrition without fibre, because it feeds your microbiome.

For the fans: the most fibre rich food source that we have at present are fresh veggies, fruit like avocados, berries, figs, artichokes, beans, green beans, lentils, nuts, and seeds.

Water

Last but not least, water is the most essential part of our body as it is 60% of it. We have to replenish this daily because we constantly lose water through urine, sweat, the air that we breathe out, and the blood women in certain periods on a monthly basis lose. Altogether this amounts to at least a litre per day. You get enough water when you eat and drink normally if you have no thirst and if your urine is colourless or very straw yellow. Dark urine can sometimes point to dehydration. If you use a litre of fluid daily through water, coffee, tea, fruit juice, or wine, next to a healthy nutritional pattern you usually have enough as a grown-up. Of course, if you play a sport or when it is hot weather you increase the need for supplementation. Children and older people often have less thirst, and they have to be reminded to drink enough during the day. It is ludicrous to advise people that you have to drink three litres of water a day. There is also something like over-hydration and you can do that knowingly or unknowingly, for instance, if your kidney function is abnormal. I have had patients who were water intoxicated and needed to come into hospital.

22 MY NUTRITIONAL TIPS

After all these years in medicine and cardiology in particular, I have made my own synthesis of my insight in nutrition and the advice that I find the best, mothers and nutritional experts underscore. There is, by the way, no nutritional advice where you cannot put any question marks or comments. You have to understand that there are parts of my advice where I do not have a hard evidence base and I am looking, just like everybody else, in this domain of scientific work and research that suits my purpose. But I do try to find a compromise that at least is safe. If it doesn't work, it is not detrimental for your health, and it has to be practical. It also has to improve your cardiovascular health, in my view. Possibly I am missing the point here, or as a Cardiologist I am talking gibberish from a nutritional point of view. Because of those arguments, I could just leave out my nutritional advice. But looking at the inconsistencies and difficulties in interpretation for people in all the scientific and popular information about diets, I wouldn't like you to remain curious about my take on this. You might find my point of view beneficial to make up your own mind. You also have to realise that my tips are not necessarily for everybody or be valuable for everybody, one individual is not the same as the other one. If I hear people talk about health and lifestyle, sometimes you hear them sigh and say "oh what is not unhealthy anymore today", or "my father-in-law smoked his whole life and he was 91" and "my dad, he never did any sports and didn't look at his food at all—he would have fried food three times a week, a big piece of cake every day, he would drink a carton of beer and died at an old age". Well, you can't argue with these comments. We are looking at the exceptions of course, those exceptions that give us an excuse.

We like to hear that you can prove everything with statistics because we can then discard them or ignore them. A classic example is that of the family with two brothers of whom one reached the age of ten and the other one 90 years of age. So both of them on average lived 50 years. If a statistic gives you weird or wrong results then that is not caused by the wrong statistic method but because the person who is making it is not a specialist, he is might not be precise in how he applied the statistics. Math and numbers are and will remain the only way to differentiate the exception of the rule. Sometimes we just read too fast and interpret the correct statistics just plain wrongly. If a disease in a country with ten million people at a certain point of time is killing 30 thousand persons because of an extra risk factor, whilst five years ago only 20 thousand persons (0.2% of the population) died of that disease, then the newspapers write in big letters correctly that the problem has increased by half (or 50%) and you can talk about a worrying evolution. But on the other hand, it is true that only 0.3% of the total population died and not 50 or 50.2%. "Increase with" is often being confused with "increased until". You shouldn't neces-sarily believe everything that is published in the newspapers and everybody knows someone who has smoked all their life and survived until old age.

The remarks that I just made were not out of my imagination, but I heard them in a pub in Kalgoorlie. I asked the lady what her dad did for a living and it seemed he was a postie his whole life and in his free time he went prospecting and hunting rabbits when he was not working in his garden. So maybe he never did any sport and maybe he did not do any of the healthy nutritional advices of today, but he was continuously moving around and busy, and he was a tall lean person. Maybe he had the advantage of healthy genes so that his intrinsic risk factors were low for starters because your metabolism and your hunger and feeling of satisfaction is also genetically determined in part. Most people who carry too much weight have to take on more energy than they need, but you also have individuals who gain weight much easier than normal. You have people who can eat whatever they want and still stay lean, so the following cardiovascular inspired nutritional advice is especially for those people who do not know if they have good genes or are exceptions to the rules.

Variation in food and trying new things

Just name me a food item and I will tell you what its disadvantages are. Whether a nutritional item is harmful depends often on the doses. The most important tip therefore is that above all, you have to eat with variation and not one thing excessively, except maybe fresh vegetables. Don't focus on just a few types of food even though they might be super-healthy in principle. Fruit for instance is full of vitamins, fibres, and anti-oxidants and I'm sure will be very healthy for you, but if you eat too much fruit, you can become obese or stay obese, especially if you take it in the form of calorie rich smoothies, juices, or cocktails. Variation also means that you do not always shop for your food in the same supermarket or shop. If you regularly shop at different places it is also a matter of spreading the risk, there could be something wrong with the production, the transport, or the packaging of the food, and it is also a great way to look for new ideas.

Don't follow a hunger diet

Quality is more important that quantity. Diets that require you starve for weeks do not work. That has been clearly shown. Not only do people on a starvation diet not continue on the diet, but they then become the victim of the famous yoyo effect, and in the end they stay heavier than when they started. Those who want to lose weight have to eat less step by step, but also switch to a healthier long-term nutritional pattern that is not an insult to their stomach and make them starve. That is of course a general advice, but it definitely is true in the case of prevention of heart and blood vessel disease and also for people who are slight to moderately overweight. Having said that, sometimes it is indicated in certain diseases that people have should follow a diet in which they have to abolish certain items or, the reverse, eat a lot of certain items. If you do this, always do it in consultation with your doctor. The same is also true for bariatric surgery. Obese people are often helped more with a stomach bypass operation than with a diet alone.

Mindful eating

With mindful eating you stay in the moment, enjoying every mouthful by eating it slowly and chewing on it well. In the meantime, you can have a nice conversation with the people at your table. Don't eat like a machine but concentrate on the tastes and aromas of what you are putting into your mouth. Experience the different textures of the food in your mouth and take a pause to eat. Don't eat behind the wheel of your car or in front of your computer. This is all going to make you more mindful about your nutrition, of the big pleasure that food can give you, but also about the quantity of the food that you are taking in.

Eat a little less

To count calories neurotically is not necessary, but most people in our society eat more than they need. Look around you. We are too fat. More than half of Australians suffer from being overweight or obese. If you would follow all of my tips regarding food, alcohol, and exercise, your body weight will slowly but surely improve and that is especially important because the wrong food and lack of exercise not only can lead to obesity but also can cause type 2 diabetes. Most scientists are in agreement that overweight and obesity—the first one you have with a BMI between 25 and 30, the second one if your BMI is higher than 30—increase the risk of the development of heart and blood vessel disease. It is of interest that people who already have congestive heart failure have in general a better prognosis if they also have obesity as compared to when they are not obese. Why, we don't know, and we call that phenomenon the obesity paradox.

Another extremely interesting research result is that people with only mild obesity do not have an increased risk of dying early and that people who are overweight but without obesity have even less risk than people with a normal or low BMI. It looks like we hear the bells' toll, but they don't exactly know where the clapper is! Maybe we should not look at the BMI that much but perhaps on the circumference on your waist in comparison to your length. More and more specialists are using your abdomen circumference measured around your waist in the space between your lower ribs and the start of your hip bone when you exhale—but without pulling your stomach in—and it should not be more than half of your height, so somebody with a big belly who otherwise is lean can have a lower BMI than a person who has a little bit of extra fat everywhere and still have a higher risk. Perhaps we should also pay more attention to risk factors associated with being overweight instead of the kilos. So for instance, the risk of developing high blood pressure is directly related to weight but there are also obese people with a normal blood pressure and lean people with hypertension. The same is true for type 2 diabetes—not everybody with a BMI over 30 or a significant enlarged abdomen has diabetes, but the statistics are very clear that your risk to develop diabetes is clearly related to the more weight you are carrying.

It is also clear nowadays that one calorie is not the same as the other calorie and that we have been hammering for a reduction of fat and fatty acids and not paying enough attention to bad carbohydrates, but it is a fact that a calorie that you do not consume can't make you grow fat. People sometimes feel compelled to finish whatever food is on their plate and even to have a second helping despite not feeling any hunger anymore. It is better to just start your meal with a portion which is just too small to satisfy your appetite, eat slowly, and then you can still have the pleasure to take a little bit extra afterwards.

Buy fresh, non-processed food

Please try to get as much non-processed food as you can. The preservatives and artificial colouring present in ready-made food are not the problem here because they are very well controlled by government regulations and in general you can eat them safely, but the kind of pre-fab products in which they are being put, often carry too much sugar, salt, trans-fatty acids, or omega 6 fatty acids, and that is definitely bad for your heart and blood vessels. In general, you can say that the more a nutritional item looks like the natural basic product and the least amount of industrial processes were used to make it, the healthier it is. For instance, filet americain or steak tartare is much better prepared freshly by yourself than to buy it already in a little can. In that way you can be responsible for determining the freshness of the steak and it is you who decides how much mayonnaise and herbs you are putting in it. Use as little additional sugars as possible.

Sugar is much more detrimental than fat

Snack on sweets as little as possible and if you can don't have candy, soft drinks, and ban foods where you have added sugar completely from your menu. That is true for commercial food that you buy ready from the shop as well as food that you prepare yourself. Sugar is a form of carbohydrates and although carbohydrates as a basic element are useful for most people you have to use carbohydrates with intelligence. Don't use refined carbohydrates which shoot your blood sugars into the stratosphere. Choose non-refined wholemeal unpeeled sources of carbohydrates systematically over white bread, white pasta, white rice, which is an important trio of stuff that makes you fat.

Carbohydrates: eat them in moderation and not in combination with a lot of fat

Fatty acids and proteins together with carbohydrates do not go well together according to many nutritional experts. In our food there are usually that many carbohydrates that the excess in energy is being stored in the body as fat. For instance, if you drink soft drinks with your meal or you take a sugar rich dessert your insulin is going to go sky high which is going to facilitate the storage of both fats and sugars. When you steer clear of bad carbohydrates you reduce the insulin production and you improve your ketosis which is the production of ketones as an alternative energy source for glucose, so if you use less carbohydrates you burn more fat. Despite scientific studies that service opposite camps, I think that whilst we are awaiting a final outcome it is sensible to steer clear of consuming large amount of carbohydrates and definitely no refined carbohydrates at all after a portion of nutrition which is rich in fat. If you would use a little portion of carbohydrates with a normal portion of fat rich food that should be alright and a bigger portion of non-refined carbohydrates with a small portion of fish or meat can work as well, but a lot of both in the same meal is not advisable according to many specialists. If, for instance, you have a big plate of wholemeal pasta with a good amount of a fatty meat sauce that is probably worse for your metabolism, your weight, and in the end your heart, than we have the same portion of pasta in the afternoon with a light fish sauce and at night a piece of meat with some salad but without a significant carbohydrate component. I am not for extreme low-carb or no carb diets that encourage people to not eat bread, pasta, rice, or potatoes. I think that a feeding pattern should also be practical. Not all people have the time or the inspiration to look every day for alternatives for bread and other traditional ways of using carbohydrates. I do like oatmeal porridge with blueberries, but after five days it is coming out of my ears! Sandwiches are usually the only item that is easily accessible to eat in many circumstances like meetings, being on the road and abroad. To never have bread is very difficult for most people to maintain and never eating pasta, rice, or potatoes does not work if you go out for a meal once in a while or visit friends for a meal. My advice therefore is do eat bread but in moderation and, if you can, have wholemeal bread. With your potatoes eat them unpeeled and use the skin in mashed potatoes as well. The insulin peak caused by carbohydrates also varies depending on the way you prepare your food. If you cook, you change the molecular structure of your nutritional item. Uncooked food like the carbohydrates in fresh fruit or in a raw carrot increases your insulin levels less than if you cook it. Slightly cooked food like pasta al dente is better than the same pasta cooked for a longer time, and to let carbohydrates cool off after you cook them and then eat them like pasta, rice, or boiled potatoes in a salad for instance, is more healthier than the same item consumed warm.

Eat the whole fruit

Fruit is very healthy and in principle you can eat whatever you like from it. But always eat the whole fruit. With the peel and all if that is possible, unprocessed and with all the fibres. Those will look after the sugar in the fruit and not boost the sugar level in your blood too much. That is why it is advisable that you do not drink industrially produced fruit juices and definitely no clear juices without any fibres. I think parents have to be responsible and teach their kids not only to drink soft drinks as little as possible, but definitely also commercial fruit juice as little as possible. Nectar drinks are a definitely a no-go. Self-made fruit juice is healthier than juice from the shop but eating the whole fruit in its natural form is always better. Berries are absolutely tops. You can eat them as much as you like. You can eat fruit separately or in combination with other healthy nutrition at any moment of the day. Only people with diabetes have to watch what type of fruit they eat because it is not good when they have fruits with too much fructose. Berries, melons, and prunes are better for them than bananas or grapes.

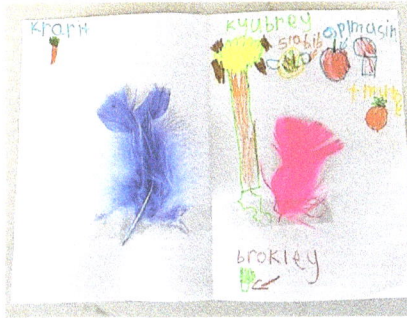

8. *This is Jeanette's idea about healthy food: carrot, broccoli, tomato and strawberry.*

Eat your veggies

Vegetables should always be the main component of your hot meal. Make sure that half of your plate is full of veggies. Veggies that you like raw should be eaten raw, but cooked vegetables are still the healthiest nutrition you can find. I prefer to eat fresh veggies or deep-frozen veggies. Vegetables are, I guess, the only nutrition which you can eat as much as you want without overdoing the calories if they are not treated with unhealthy products. Also take into consideration what I said before, you have variation in your food and that you don't eat a lot of a single item. You should also realise that not only potatoes and corn but also turnips and items like beans and lentils contain quite a bit of carbohydrates.

23 EAT AS LITTLE BAD FATS AS POSSIBLE

Be careful talking to carbo-phobia people that preach that you can eat as much fat as you want as long as you don't take in any carbohydrates! To live in extremes is never good for you and whoever eats a lot of fat will probably also get too many trans-fatty acids and omega 6 fatty acids and will therefore increase the risk of becoming obese, getting heart and blood vessel disease, and type 2 diabetes. However, fats are much less bad for you as we thought before. Of the so-called "good fats" like the ones in nuts, olive oil, avocados, or fatty fish, you can eat whatever you want. But the trans-fatty acids and omega 6 fats you have to restrain and try and avoid them altogether. With fat in meat you can have another tip here—you can fry meat by putting it in hot coconut oil which seems to be the best compromise.

Do not eat industrially prepared meat products. Go for untouched biodynamic grown meat and keep the so-called charcuterie sausages and other industrially made meat products far from you because they often contain sugars, bad fats, and refined carbohydrates. Most people eat too much meat anyway so why not choose an alternative once in a while. You do not have to eat meat every day. During the seven days of your week you can, for instance, have a day with hard-boiled eggs or an omelet instead of meat, perhaps a day with champignons or another replacement for the meat, a day with fish, a day with crustaceans, a day with chicken, and then the last two days you can happily eat some cow or pork. When you choose your meat go for quality—preferably from animals that were bred in a biodynamic way, not only because that is nicer for the animal but also because those animals themselves enjoyed a much better feeding pattern. And yes, it often costs a little bit more money however with less meat consumption you might break even but you improve your health.

Dairy

Dairy is a difficult one. One person copes with the use of dairy better than the other. Studies looking at potential pros and cons of different types of dairy with fat or half fat or skim or A2 or A1 and A2 are very contradictory at times. The good thing is that you can pretty simply find out whether certain dairy products are good for you by trying them for a couple of weeks and then figure out whether you have side effects. If you really enjoy yoghurt and cheese, then in any case go for the raw product without additional sugars or funny tastes.

Drink plenty of water

You can drink water, tea, herbal tea, coffee, self-pressed fruit juice (one glass per day), and a maximum of two standard drinks of alcohol (and really only one for women). To pimp your water, you can add some citrus or sugar free syrup. If you take a zero-calorie juice, then it is probably healthier than a normal soft drink with sugar. However, with the 'zero' stuff, I would be careful. The notion that the sugar replacement aspartame causes cancer has no scientific basis but there is a different type of danger. There are good studies to suggest that all these products without sugars or replacement sugars increase your appetite for sugar which means that you will eat more and in the end get more sugar and calories than when you would have taken normal cola or tonic. According to some studies zero drinks and diet drinks would increase the risk of developing metabolic syndrome and type 2 diabetes. The use of these products does not lower but increases the risk. As per usual these studies are observational studies which show that A and B are found together but not necessarily prove that they are the cause of each other. The conclusion for me therefore, is that we don't know exactly how it works but there is enough evidence to be very careful with the usage of these drinks. Of course, always drinking only water, coffee, or tea is not something that people aspire to. My favourite non-alcoholic beverage is one third of home-pressed grapefruit or orange juice with two thirds fizzy water, and of course once in a while a glass of wine...

Breakfast

It is better not to have breakfast than to have a bad breakfast. Whether a breakfast is really the most important meal of the day is a discussion that we will leave alone. Maybe that is also an often heard but without base type of statement. I think that breakfast can be a very good start to the day if it contains proteins, good fats, and fibre rich non-refined carbohydrates like all fruits, but I think that you better give your breakfast away if it were bread with chocolate spread or something else sweet, and definitely not sugared fat-free yoghurt and mueslis, pancakes with sugar and other refined carbohydrates. Don't get fooled by commercial breakfast cereals which scream on the packaging they have extra vitamins or perhaps some pieces of dried fruit. If they are made from refined carbohydrates or have added sugars they are not to be used.

Be happy to have a snack before you go to bed. One of the other dogmas that you shouldn't eat anything at night time or maybe only some celery because you don't move at night and therefore all the calories that you eat at night would be transformed into extra body weight. Well indeed, having a heavy meal late at night before you go to bed is not recommended because it will interfere with your sleep which is important. That is the same if you eat a big amount of fruit or vegetables that have a lot of vitamin C. If you have a protein rich snack like a hardboiled egg or a chicken leg or piece of cheese at night, hey, it is nice, it satisfies your appetite, and I don't think it would harm you.

You have to give in once in a while

I think one of the important things when you talk about nutrition, is moderation, and that implies that once in a while you can do things which are different. So if every couple of weeks you have a nice piece of cake or you are at a party and you enjoy some of the food they have there, if it is possible to not have those items for the rest of the time, then I think go ahead and enjoy.

Also, importantly, deal with your emotional problems and mental health.

To eat, dear reader, is a much bigger part of our life, our brain, and our society, than just having some nutrition or the taste of some nutrition. The life of wild animals only revolves around finding and consuming food. To find food and to digest it is their most important task for the day. And for humans, for hundreds of thousands of years that was the case. It is only since the hunter gatherer became farmers that we had more influence on our food situation, but the daily struggle for life and especially for getting fat, went on deep into the 18th century for most western Europeans, and today that is still the case in a large part of the world. Because evolution is slow, our brain is still tuned to getting food although most people in the rich countries don't have to worry about it or spend a lot of time on it. Okay, we do work for our food but an Australian family on average spends less than 30% of their budget on food. Still, we are conscious or unconsciously busy with gathering food. It is important for our daily rhythm and one of our most important social activities in our family and friends. Because we can afford it, we have made a whole culture of gastronomy etiquette and that is only getting "worse"—the tsunami of cookbooks, TV chefs, and eating programs is amazing.

Nature designed our bodies to get hungry and like food. As we need nutrition, we like food in order to be motivated to eat! To like something is a form of pleasure and pleasure has to do with emotions. Therefore, consuming food is—without realizing it—an emotionally and psychologically important activity. It is no wonder that people with emotional problems often as a compensation mechanism or as a reward system, eat abnormally. They will have periods where they eat abnormally a lot, or they become anorexic, or they become alcoholic. To consume food not only fills our stomach but also our brain and before you know it, you are in a vicious cycle. Psychological problems can make us eat the wrong things, and because we eat the wrong things we get more heart and vascular disease, we become fat, we get other problems with our body, we feel worse and therefore we eat even more unhealthy stuff. Maybe we should take more time to look at our heart and ask the question honestly whether we need some help in our soul.

We currently live in a time and society with big mental problems. We have never had so much material wealth and we never had such a lot of mental illness. Behind the doors of our beautiful homes and modern apartments we have a lot of tragedy. Broken relationships, lonely people , more and more kids are being diagnosed with ADHD or another psychological condition, our suicides go up, and we lose ourselves in a parallel universe where we have fake versions of people that we meet who have a less and less eye for what is really happening inside the human being. The taboo on admitting or having psychological problems is really big and a lot of us humans have no social network in which people are interested in us or really love us. We don't have people that give us a pat on the back and look out for us to see whether we are okay and help us with our problems. There-fore, if you are worried about your heart but you also struggle with being overweight, underweight, with your fitness and your health, your health in general, please talk to people. Talk about it with your partner, with a good friend, with your GP, with your kids, with a psychologist or psychiatrist, it serves no purpose to go from one diet adventure into another diet adventure if you don't address the root of your problem. That is why in the beginning of the book I stated that it is so important to have a little walk every day. Walking in nature helps people to clear the mind and to just take a step back from all the struggles of daily life. It will enable you to put things in a different perspective. Maybe adjust your ambitions and maybe come to the conclusion that you need professional help. Everybody has periods when they are under enormous pressure and we don't talk about it with anybody. When we have the flu or a toothache, then we want to have that solved straight away and you are right, but if we have prob-lems with our feeling or thoughts then we wait forever before we ask for help. Heart and blood vessel disease also occurs in people who are balanced and generally happy, but often these diseases are fuelled from our computer, our brain, and when you read this maybe this is also the case for you.

Don't give diabetes a chance

One third of people with increased weight will suffer from type 2 diabetes. 50% of them develop more physical complaints earlier or later and those complaints are usually heart and blood vessel prob-lems. When you eat carbohydrates your blood sugar level goes up. After a couple of hours it drops down to its normal level under the influence of insulin which is being produced in your pancreas. In people with diabetes, that system does not work well, and the sugar level stays too high. Type 2 diabetes, which is approximately 90% of all diabetes, is usually developed over the years and type 1 diabetes usually starts in children, but it can happen later on in life as well. In any case, in the body of type 2 diabetes there is too little insulin, and it does not react sufficiently on the insulin still being produced. People with type 1 diabetes are not making insulin at all. At first you don't notice that you have type 2 diabetes, but then you start to get symptoms like you have to drink a lot of water, you have to pass a lot of urine, you get a dry mouth, your sight is getting bad, you get constipation, you get itchy, little traumas or little wounds that you get are not healing properly, you are tired, you lose weight. If your type 2 diabetes is not controlled, then your fat metabolism is out of kilter and you have a higher risk of getting chronic infections. That process can damage your blood vessels and you get accelerated atherosclerosis. This is the reason why people with diabetes have a higher risk of suffering from a heart attack, a myocardial infarction, congestive heart failure, or a stroke. In women with diabetes that risk is even higher than in men. Those who suffer from diabetes have to pay special attention to the risks for cardiovascular disease and have to be careful not to place all the complaints they have on the diabetes, and the latter is also true for doctors. Type 2 diabetes by the way, can be treated very well. Medication, but also healthy feeding patterns, nutrition without refined carbohydrates in combination with a lot of physical exercise can do miracles and one nice example is that in people that underwent bariatric surgery when the risk of diabetes or if diabetes was present, the abolishing of diabetes is sometimes like a miracle.

24 DON'T JUST ACCEPT THAT YOU HAVE A GENETIC CONDITION CAUSING HEART OR BLOOD VESSEL DISEASE

If you are born in a family where there are a lot of heart problems, then the risk is real that you may have to deal with the same issues. It can be related to a bad lifestyle that will be transferred from one generation to another, like if your parents smoked or had a lot of candies, then the risk is you think it is normal behaviour, as well as having the previously mentioned genetic factors. Your predisposition for a genetic disease is something you cannot prevent but secondary prevention, which means to recognize the problems quickly or actively look for them, can be very worthwhile for many genetic abnormalities. It is important to check with brothers, sisters, parents, grandparents, or your uncles and aunts whether they have died from heart or blood vessel disease or a cardiac arrest. Also, whether there is high blood pressure, cholesterol problems, peripheral vascular disease, and all these types of issues. Maybe you could draw up a genetic tree of life of your family. If you find two or three of those cases, then maybe this is something you can discuss with your GP. He would be the person to discuss whether it would be useful to look for a genetic abnormality. GPs with a lot of experience who have seen families for many years will see certain abnormalities repeat themselves. Still, they don't think to discuss these other genetic factors or familial problems with them every time somebody from their family comes with a problem like a cold or a rash.

I don't know the exact figures for Australia but in the United Kingdom they think more than 600,000 people are walking around with one or more defective genes which cause an increased risk of heart attacks or another genetic heart disease. That is almost 1:100 persons, so when there is a suspicion of having a genetically determined or otherwise risk of heart disease, your doctor can look for hidden symptoms or can have a genetic test done to look for gene mutations in your DNA, at least as far as science is able to do that today. Hypertrophic cardiomyopathy, Marfan syndrome, and Brugada syndrome are examples of hereditary abnormalities in which we are very knowledgeable about the genetic factors. Of other genetic abnormalities, we do know that they are hereditary, but we don't know the exact cause, or we may have an idea, but it seems that there are multiple mutations playing a role. Genetic cardiology is a specialty that is booming and in 2016 British scientists developed a new and cheaper test that can find a big group of genes that are known to be part of hereditary heart disease in one go. In Australia, genetic tests are only paid by health insurance if they happen in a recognized centre and you have to realize that a genetic test does include risks because our knowledge of the genes is evolving faster than treatments for these genetic abnormalities. The test person probably needs a good psychological support mechanism before and after such an investigation. By the way, I am not a fan of the DNA tests that you can do through an internet kit. For starters, those kits are not always reliable but also the interpretation of are not very accurate. It is not only that you could have a certain mutation meaning you will automatically get the disease, but where that mutation plays a role, and even if and when that might happen. With most hereditary diseases we find at least more than one factor involved which makes it more complicated.

In any case, genetic investigations will be more and more important, that evolution is unstoppable. There are many persons who after a genetic testing will pave the way to making 'designer babies' and that we may go on a path where we know so many things about ourselves, our partners, and our potential children that we really don't want to know. People with genetic risks will perhaps have more abortions or not have in vitro fertilization embryos implanted if they don't like the genetic test results. As an optimist, I don't think genetic testing will be misused on a big scale like this. People also opposed our laws on euthanasia for a long time and we have managed to be very reasonable in this 'hot item' at present. It is up to the bioethics professionals to carefully assess what is happening in our society today and how we can ethically use all these opportunities that science gave us.

Suggestions for prevention for policy makers and people that use policy makers (voters)

People are getting older without doing anything but do not always stay healthy. I would like to end this maintenance book about some of my suggestions for our policy makers, our financial planning, and some remarks about our change in psychology during COVID-19 which is the time I was writing this in 2020. Our country has a healthcare system which is the envy of many countries in the world, so it can't be that bad. I will suggest some concrete ideas with respect to cardiovascular prevention a little bit later which will pay the initial investment back very quickly.

Every year on the 1st January we wish each other not only Happy New Year but also good health. We find nothing as important as good health, and we state that very often. Politicians should have that simple notion always in their eyesight, even more than any other challenge to our society. It is time for a radical change in the world. We as a society are dealing with health and medical science, and that starts already in utero. We should teach our kids that they are responsible for their bodies themselves, both physical and mental health, and that it is better to prevent problems than to have to go to doctors to solve them. That is of course a cliché to some but in real life, the education of our children rarely focuses on prevention of health problems. One way that hasn't worked is by abolishing physical health classes in many schools. Because we live in a rich country with many active doctors and many people would rather take pills—whether they are prescribed or over the counter—than make themselves tired with exercise to prevent bad health.

The risk of over consumption of medication is a real one. Some health economics groups wish to exclude the population from receiving medical checks until they have proven to be sick. However, I believe this is too late as these problems can be prevented by educating them to live a healthier lifestyle. It is true that we are very quickly and perhaps too quickly seeking help from medication, but the rest of the health economics logic is BS. It is not intelligent to assume that you are healthy until you are obviously not healthy. You just can't tell whether any random person is healthy. In healthy looking people, you can find a time bomb or a slowly deteriorating process, and there-fore people would be much better off to go and see a doctor regularly for a check-up. The chance is very real that doing this will mean less medication and less disease, which also means less cost to society and the health budget. So instead of waiting until you get symptoms that the doctor then has to try to get rid of, it is sensible to have preventa-tive investigations at certain times to check whether you are healthy and, if it is the case that you are still healthy, to check whether you are still on the right path to stay healthy.

Almost anything in our "social healthy state" can be checked and double-checked on known or hypothetical risks. We send inspectors to check up on our usually very well-functioning teachers, we have our cars checked technically, we look at our buildings and check them for fire risk, and we put CCTV cameras everywhere to discourage and catch vandalism and crime, but if we discuss our health, something that every 1st January we think is one of the most important resolutions we have, we are expected to solve the problems when they occur. So if there is one area you can reduce risks and negative consequences by early prevention, then that must be in the area of health.

They calculated in the Netherlands in 2016 that smoking was costing the society there—which is a similar size as Australia—11 billion euros, whilst the net income out of the taxes of the smoking articles was giving the state 2 billion euros. The cost of smoking every year is 950 billion euros worldwide, which is an incomprehensible amount of money.

Cardiovascular disease costs the US one billion dollars on medical expenses and loss of productivity per day! We do get sick at a certain point in time but in that case, we are collectively, including the government, like an ostrich with their head in the sand. "Ah it won't be anything," we say to ourselves, "tomorrow it will be okay, it will go away". Does that mean with any little pain or problem you have to rush to the doctor? Of course not, but you do have to recognize important alarm signals and regularly see a health professional with or without complaints. You see, to live long or healthy is not a natural automatic given.

To explore this a bit further, I will just go back to the basics of life and biology. Consciously or unconsciously a lot of people just assume that being healthy is our normal biological standard program, and that our bodies are designed to have an average of 80 years. That is not true. Every individual form of life from bacterium A to whale Z are genetically programmed to pass on its genetic material but how much time that form of life has to actually accomplish that is irrelevant for the cosmos. We are still not sure what were the circumstances that started life on earth approximately 4.3 billion years ago, but what we do know is that all forms of life are temporary packages of molecules and atoms that have to work hard their whole life long to get energy and to defend themselves against harmful influences from the outside. At least until the moment that they can replicate themselves, otherwise they just disappear. As soon as you have your offspring, it is not any more detrimental from a biological point of view if you are falling apart in the atoms and chemicals that built you in the first place. Organisms usually get to the age that their environment allows them to be. As evolution thought that you might need wings, camouflage colours, a big body or a top IQ then the chance that you are eating is larger than you are being eaten, and therefore you can live longer than comparable sorts of life that do not have those defensive characteristics. If that is not the case then your life will be shorter and it doesn't matter, as long as you are spreading your DNA. Therefore, there is no real law about the duration that life forms live. That can vary from some ten minutes to some thousands of years. There is discussion about both extremes because it is not always clear when life starts. Are you counting the phase in the egg or larvae as life? Or when it stops? When does a tree die, for instance? Dolania americana is a one-day fly that is born, has copulation, and dies within 30 minutes. Endoliths are organisms that live in stone and they can stay there for over ten thousand years. There is also a big difference in life expectancy between vertebrae animals. Some little crawfish live less than a month. The Greenland shark however will take 150 years to be ready to copulate and can reach an age of 400 years. Among mammals, we are on the top of the chain followed by elephants. I just want to make the point that from a nature/biology basis, you are not required to live a long time.

The way in which evolution manifests itself is fascinating and shows you many ingenious solutions to our problems. And that is why we get the impression that there is a master plan behind all this, but until now no master has declared itself. If a master did exist, its goals or decision criteria are pretty random to me. He doesn't seem to have biological or evolutionary tools that can improve the quality or the quantity of lifeforms to a higher level. The creations are in constant interaction with each other and with cosmic and earth forces of nature. Luck and chaos are often influential. One tsunami or one meteorite from the skies and we can redo everything. If that is a so-called master plan, then there are serious shortcomings. Different species and individuals come and go but the earth is always there, or at least for a couple of billion years. I will leave it to the philosophers to find out whether life has a deeper meaning, but if we have a task to fulfil on earth then it is definitely not one to get old.

We think that we would like to get old because we have evolved into intelligent and social human beings. We have long term relationships, and we think it a waste that our knowledge and experience get lost when life stops. We think about our future and our place in the cosmos and we realise that we have mortality. Maybe this last item is the only thing that really separates us from other animals. If we want to live longer then it is necessary for our biological task to have good genes and luck that no bad omen happens to us. But we have to work on that to make it happen.

It is not because in western society people are on average now 80 years of age that every person reaches that age because he just eats and drinks healthily and doesn't put his car against a tree. Our life expectancy is the sum of all the measures that we have taken as people to have our kids go safely through the first critical days of life and so able to stretch out our life expectancy far beyond the point where we have given our genes to the next generation. Part of your personal life expectancy is in your genes, feeding pattern, and educa-tion, but as people grow up to be adults and make their own choices, they can take more and more responsibility for their health. I think this is important to realise because Mother Nature didn't give us a guarantee for having a long life. She has, through evolution given women the ability to bear children after the age of 15. Every two to three years, she could give a newborn baby between one to three years of breastfeeding, and at times we did that and some populations in nature still do that. In fact, the World Health Organisation promotes it. In the period of breastfeeding, women are less fertile. In any case, by reaching around 40 years of age we have been on earth long enough to put three to four kids into the world and to bring them to maturity so they can have children themselves. In this way both mother and father have replicated themselves and the extra kids are just there to compensate possible children's death.

In the 1800s, child death was 43%. So, from a biological viewpoint your task is done when you are around 40. Maybe it is a coincidence but as from 40, muscle strength, regeneration ability, hearing, and sight, goes downhill and with women, fertility. Some degeneration processes start earlier. For instance, the big arteries in your body start to get atherosclerosis in your 30s. Also, from an intellectual point of view you are over the hill from around 25 years of age. Okay, even in the middle ages there were people that reached 70 or 80 years without the medical knowledge of today. But those who want to live long and healthy and not completely depend on luck, genetic presence, or fast reflexes in driving a car on the Mitchell Freeway has to learn to look after his body, as a car enthusiast looks after his old timers. It is not good enough to just paint over rusty spots and put wax on your car. What is underneath the hood in the engine deserves much more attention because indeed we are much more focused on the exterior signs of decay. We hate that we get little wrinkles, that we get sagging breasts and bellies, and that we go bald, and we forget that the inside of our body is getting old exactly the same as the outside.

The bottom line is that people are getting older, but they might not stay healthy. Doctors and patients are much better off not to wait until people get in their 50's and 60's and get problems. We need a plan!

25 PREVENTIVE MEDICAL EXAMINATION EVERY SIX YEARS IS ADVISABLE

My suggestion is that people have a free psychological/medical investigation when they have Medicare benefits around every six years or maybe more often if there are questions or problems detected in the meantime. This way the government will be sure that all eligible Australians would go for these medical examinations. Of course, during childhood there are already plenty of investigations that happen preventatively by their GP and in early childcare. There is also a scheme for immunizations and dental care included in these check-ups for children. I think these investigations and immunization schemes are very important and helpful but are not going far enough. We would need to use these moments to check all important physical, psychological, and social factors, and to discuss those issues that are important for the child at that time.

We need to then use this information and follow through as they grow up to be an adolescent and into adulthood. Who should carry this out? I suggest it should not only be the doctor but a team including parents, teachers and other key people in the education and mentoring of the child.

When the child turns six or seven, early childhood is finished, and the child will enter a completely new world. They will have tasks, and responsibilities, and there will be expectations when they go to school. This is a perfect opportunity to check whether the physical and psychological progression of the child is in keeping with what we would expect from a child that age. Furthermore, the child could be educated in healthy food and nutrition, dental hygiene, the importance of sport and physical exercise, and to teach them about their own physical and spiritual integrity. The whole wellbeing of the child is the focal viewpoint. We can then also talk about the dangers of traffic, of the possibilities and risk of social media, and imaging screens like computers and TV. We can discuss what is normal and not normal in the social dealings with each other as children and with their interactions with grownups. Here you can tackle issues like bullying, the intrusion of privacy, grooming, physical violence, psychological violence, sexual predators, or even worse forms of behaviour of which children can be the victim. Doctors and other trusted persons can have a crucial role in that part of their development.

When the child turns 11 or 12, we can prepare boys and girls for puberty. It is around this time that girls will get their first period, both sexes will kiss for the first time, they may get into pornography sites on the computer and start to experience the 'manipulations' of the Internet like Facebook, Twitter and the like. It is time to discuss differences and similarities between genders, how to have relationships, how to use contraception methods, and how to protect against cervical cancer and pregnancy. We also need to discuss the use of legal and illegal drugs and the specific risks of alcohol and drugs on the heart as well as the rest of the body. This is also a good time to start with lessons on CPR and other essential first aid techniques. It would be fantastic for no pupil to leave our education system without recognizing symptoms of a heart attack or a stroke or to be able to do CPR. At this time, their doctor could take their first electrocardiograph to find possible congenital heart abnormalities. However, this might be best to wait until they are 14 because then it is easier to differentiate between the electrocardiogram of a not completely grown up heart and a grown-up heart.

Children who participate in intensive sports and therefore have extra risks in case of a hidden heart problem do not usually start these types of sport before the age of 14. It is also useful at that age to look at the physical features of the child to see how grown up they actually are because at this age, especially in boys, there is often a big variation. Some boys of 14 still have a child's body, others have lots of muscles, big bones, and their voice is breaking. For competition sports it could be a reason to have children practice their sport in a younger age category because that might improve their physical and mental integrity. Fourteen years of age is also the age when children will experience their sexual preferences. They start to masturbate, they make love with each other, they start love relationships, and they get hold of cigarettes, alcohol, cannabis, or other drugs. What they already learn about these issues when they were 12 has to be repeated and be brought up to date. They also need to be comfortable to ask questions about it. They need to be aware of the most important sexually transmitted diseases. They need to know how to use a condom and the contraception pill, and they need to know what to do to prevent an unwanted pregnancy or, if it happened, where to go and what to do and what the options are.

The fifth medical examination in one's life could be done when they are legally seen as a grown-up. They are 18-years of age and they may go to university or TAFE, start work, and they will get into a different, more competitive environment. They will see different opportunities, but they will also have the ability to follow temptations. At this stage it is important that they understand what their body and mind can take and what it cannot. The doctor can also check what their vaccine status is, take a second ECG, and he can educate them with reading material, videos and websites for them to get information about their health. They are able to drive a car, they may be a leader in the sports club, they will travel without their parents, they are leaving the protection and the care of their home to go and live somewhere else; all beautiful reasons to refresh their knowledge of medical emergencies and first aid, so that they can help themselves and others.

The sixth investigation is around the age of 24-years of age. A lot of young adults have finished university, they have found a profession, or they are looking for a job. Usually they have a partner, they are thinking of having a family, and they need the elementary knowledge and skills to deal with pregnancy and babies. They also need to know about healthy lifestyle not only to give their kids a good basis but also for their own health. So now they are getting into the period where they have to make it. That they want to be professionally successful. They need to learn to balance work time and private time and that balance will be under tremendous pressure as the years go by. That is definitely the case when the first baby is born. In the meantime, their body is going slowly but surely downhill. In their mid-20s people who have never had problems before start thinking about how different parts of their body are functioning. They must realise that being healthy is not a given any more and they must take their lifestyle and wellbeing into their own hands because nobody else other than perhaps their partner will motivate them to do that. They should also go for a health check every six years at the age of 30, 36, 42, etc. if their wish is to have continuing health.

I have made a small schedule with tips that you could follow in your adult life or which you could perhaps add to your health plan. Of course, as a Cardiologist my emphasis is on cardiovascular health, but GPs and other specialists could put their own priorities as well as I do on these moments of preventative medicine. In this way you would have certain points in your lifetime to check for not only cardiovascular disease but all kinds of cancers like colon cancer, breast cancer, problems with menopause, erectile dysfunction, osteoporosis, eye problems, metabolic diseases like diabetes, or you could be able to detect dementia early.

In your 20s

Choose a GP who lives in your neighbourhood and who you feel comfortable forming a relationship with. It is important that you can talk to your physician and that he or she knows you and your lifestyle over a period of time. That means that you have to discuss your lifestyle honestly with them. Ask your doctor to check your weight, blood pressure, cholesterol, heartbeat, and blood sugars, this way you have a good basis on which to check later changes. Be sure to keep your body moving. A lot of people in their 20s stop playing sports after their school years, but it is easier to be active in your middle ages if you never stop it in the first place. Don't smoke or drink unless in moderation. Pregnant women must check their weight and blood sugars.

In your 30s

Be aware that you and your family are living a healthy life. Kids often copy their parents' lifestyle knowingly or unconsciously whether they like it or not. So do give your kids a good basis and avoid patterns of possible bad habits which you will have learned from your parents. Make it a habit to eat healthily with the whole family and to walk a lot, play sport, live outdoors, be active, maybe owning a dog would be something to consider as this would promote all these moving activities, and it is also good for the kids' immunity build-up. Grow your own vegetables, have some chickens, in this case the kids can understand and realise and taste the value of fresh food. Be in charge of your level of stress. People in their 30s are often slaves to their work and even brag about how busy they are. In this way they feel important which is BS. Don't do it. Do take and plan time for yourself and for your family. Your parents are still alive, and they are mentally okay, so this is also a good time to check what kind of illnesses were in your family. You can then discuss it with your GP.

And then you are in your 40s

We are halfway through our life and we realise more than ever that we have to enjoy life, but that only can happen if you are okay between your ears! Do enjoy this glass of wine and this dinner but keep track of your belly size. This is also the phase of your life that your belly is going to drop. Your metabolism is getting slower and you have to adjust for this by eating less and eating more healthily and staying active. Because your kids are now in puberty and they are doing one hundred and one things at the same time, and perhaps because you are still very busy at work yourself it seems to you that the time is not there to move and be active. Why don't you become a member of a sporting club or have a deal with other people to go and do a sport together? I am sure that you can use this extra motivation. Have your blood sugars and blood pressure checked at least once a year and, if you find that you are snoring more or louder, do get a check for the presence of obstructive sleep apnoea. One in five adults has a form of sleep apnoea and that is dangerous for your heart so go and see your doctor.

And then you are in your 50s

You are already doing the most important tip in this phase of your life by reading this book. Inform yourself about the first symptoms of heart and blood vessel disease. Be sure that you understand the signs and symptoms of angina pectoris or a brain infarct. It is very possible that you are also taking medications perhaps for high blood pressure or cholesterol levels. Make sure you do this. Be alert for possible side effects and discuss them regularly with your doctor.

And now you are over 60!

Continue to be mobile and exercise, even when you are a cardiac patient. In the meantime, you have some grandchildren, why don't you follow them with their hobbies. It keeps you young. Haven't been cycling for donkey's years? Well, get a bicycle, perhaps an electric one, and use it for short distances. If you are still smoking or do you have pain in your calf muscles when you go for a walk? Then definitely go and have your ankle-arm index measured. Also keep an extra eye on your weight now you are needing less calories but be aware of being underweight as well as overweight. Drink at least a litre of water a day, also in wintertime. Seniors do not drink enough. If your GP gets older together with you then you know each other very well and at least the doctor has experience. That's fine. But if you notice that you are going backwards while you are still following all the advice you get then it could be of value to ask for a second opinion from a younger doctor perhaps. As patients and their doctors get older, they are more likely to do what they always did, and they have less of an eye on changes or new strategies. Even if you have a partner or a good family, it is important to prevent depression and loneliness after you stop working. This means you need to become a member of a cultural, sport or other hobby organisation. In this way you make new contacts and friends. Volunteer work could also be a great option to stay awake, not only mentally but also keeping you young at heart and enjoying a large social network. The social network is important for days that you do not have a birthday or a public holiday.

Stimulate patients to take responsibility for their health and stimulate doctors to think maximally about prevention

The pressure on the health budget is greater year by year, especially because our population is getting older. We should not look at this as fate or an evolution that is doomed to make our health system unattainable. On average we are getting older thanks to medical progress, so our government as well as the doctors have to do everything that they can to enable seniors to live those extra years as healthily as possible. There is a point where we have to teach people at a young age which aspects of their health that they cannot influence but can still monitor.

People should carry their responsibility and be able to realise the consequences of their actions. I am not talking about giving access to healthcare to only well-informed people doing the right thing, that would be inhuman and not social. But people who don't want to listen and do not try to stop smoking, for instance, even when they have bypass surgery, have to understand that the community and the government is not prepared to pay for all costs until they are dead. I believe specialists and medical ethics should think about the model to stimulate those types of patients to still take action. I do think that if we inform our population better and give them (financial!) advantages if they undergo preventive investigations at certain times during their life, and if they are trying to do the right thing with the advice that they get, that they qualify for financial rebates. By the same token, perhaps doctors should get better pay if they are more successful keeping patients healthier for longer and when their patients need less treatment.

Healthcare is working on these issues but in many cases, we are still doing exactly the opposite. The slower we are in intervening in illness, the more the doctor has to see the patient and the more they have to do so, the more they earn. Perhaps it is better if the practice of medicine is completely dependent on healthcare, so in that way medicine would only be that part of our health system that we need when the prevention plan we initiated with our patient fails for whatever reason. To organize such a plan is of course teamwork, and in this day and age doctors should not be working as individuals. In our 21st century starting your career as a solo doctor is a disaster. It is a disaster for your work/home balance if you want to see enough patients to get experience, but it is also a bad idea if you look for continuation of care, and I feel this is true for both specialists and GPs. Medical science is changing so fast and patients are often so aware of their problems that you as a doctor need a colleague to discuss cases to check out your own doubts about a problem, to be available for your patients, and to take care that people don't make mistakes or go the wrong way. I think the government doesn't have to discourage solo practices, but they should stimulate group practices.

Give people who play a sport a medical rebate and start a centre point for cardiac arrest during sport activities

Every month we read or see on television that again somewhere in Australia somebody doing sport died from a cardiac event and whether this was during a training episode, during a game, or during a mass event like a City to Surf run. This is dramatic for at least two reasons. Firstly, it is a drama for the victim of course but also for his family, friends, and the people in the club. Secondly, every time it happens there is a public outcry, especially when the victim is a child, a teenager, or young adult. Parents of children in that sport are bewildered when they read something in the newspaper about somebody that died young, and some people even start to think that doing sports is dangerous. Of course, the opposite is true. The importance of moving and physical activity to prevent diseases or to bring diseases to light, and even to treat diseases, is very important and cannot be emphasized enough. After all, if you are always sitting in your nice chair you never know how you are deteriorating. When you never play sport of course, you cannot die during sports, but the risk that you die suddenly anyway is ten times higher than when you play a sport. Only people that survive you and your family members are wondering "oh, but why didn't we know that this person had a hidden heart problem". People often have the impression that a sport-related sudden cardiac death is a rare event, and that is not completely true. Actually, we don't know how often it occurs because we don't have a good registration system. The problem is that Cardiologists are very well-trained in detecting cardiovascular problems in young people or people that want to take up sports, but on average their expertise in looking at risk for muscles or joints or the skeleton or the brain is not so good. They are also not very good at looking into all the risk factors for each of the many sports that people are doing. GPs who haven't taken up sports medicine would face the same problem, so it is important that we have a system where people that want to or already do play sports get checked by somebody who is a specialist in the field, somebody who has studied sports medicine. They would be in the perfect position to assess people's risks. These types of test could carry a rebate under our Medicare system. When we have an important part of our population checked that way, it would also reduce our overall costs because these tests would bring to light other health problems that were there but not necessarily noticed previously.

I am not the only doctor or scientist who has this opinion. In 2015 in the European Journal of Preventive Cardiology there was a whole article written about the subject of medical checks in sports, and registration of particular problems that occur during sports like sudden cardiac death. Perhaps with our modern technology (have a look at our COVID app) and website technology where it is easy to do reporting, we could find a way to have those incidents measured by witnesses, referees, trainers, doctors, etc. collating all the cases so we can investigate what happened. In this way we would not only know more about sport-related problems like sudden cardiac death, but we could also help family members of victims and informing family members about potential risks as well.

And then there are the finances. For many of us when we start our career, we spend most of our money buying a home, although for some people it is a car. When we start a family or when we invest in homes and cars, that is when our career starts, and we need to consider our financial situation. Those of us who are successful and make more money might even need a financial planner to organise their superannuation and to help them to manage their affairs in such a way that they don't have any financial hardship in the future. What is often overlooked is one's health style. When people are looking into their finances, they might look into their day to day income, their job security, and their career path opportunities. If they are very "switched on" they might realise that a divorce is very expensive, that kids can be very expensive depending on which school they go to, and that the tax man doesn't forget you! You might discuss strategies to invest your money in shares or in property or not at all and put it under your mattress, but in all those cases you assume that you are alive. Not only that you are alive but also that you are healthy because most people assume that they are born healthy and stay healthy. What I have tried to explain in the previous chapters is that health is something we have to actively pursue. So I feel that when you are doing your financial planning you also should include the management of your health because if you don't have health your financial needs might dramatically change. I give that food for thought. In 2018, we-in collaboration with Troy Macmillan from TWD (Perth and Sydney) and Mark Bell from Harvest Taxation (Perth)- got recognised for this by the financial world.

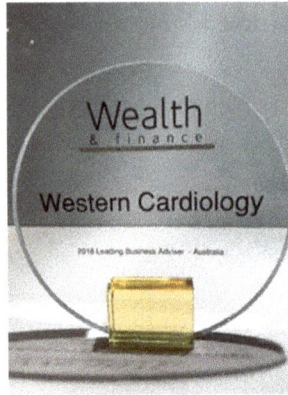

9

Last but not least, educate your doctor. We can, dear reader, do a lot ourselves as an individual and as society together. When you take your destiny in your own hands that also means that you cannot blindly follow the capacity or the dedication of your doctor. As I mentioned in previous chapters, you do have to follow a certain treatment plan long enough to give it a fair chance to work, but if you get the impression that your health is deteriorating whilst your doctor has no explanation for that or doesn't come with new suggestions then perhaps you should smell a rat and ask for a second opinion or find another doctor. Doctors have studied for at least seven years and are obliged to continuously educate themselves to follow the advances in their chosen field of specialization. That means they are without any doubt the best point to discuss your health, but it does not mean that doctors are infallible or that they are the only place where you can have a discussion. The days people just had to do what the doctor said has long gone. Be alert, do ask questions, and talk about your doubts. In other words, start a real partnership with your doctor.

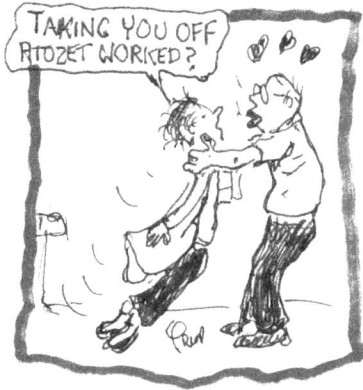

10

Share this responsibility for your health. Respect your doctor for his knowledge but also dare to challenge him to prove why he is worth it. If you feel that a GP or specialist is not doing enough to explain what your problem is, then I think you should make that a point of discussion. More and more doctors do not take enough time to inform the patients properly. A lack of satisfying and effective communication in our practices and in our hospitals is one of the biggest problems in current health care. I have seen that everywhere. Of course, it is caused by a lack of time in the way we have financially organised our healthcare, to explain things to people is not very well paid, but still it is one of the most important things that the doctor can do. Although our technology and our improved diagnostic and therapeutic guidelines are the headlines in medicine, it is still the communication skills and the ability to have a good relationship between the doctor and the patient. This ensures the patient feels like he is dealing with a trustworthy partner in that relationship—that is the difference between an excellent and a less excellent doctor. To be able to listen and to let people finish their stories during a consultation is essential. I also draw quite a bit during consultations when I have to explain to a patient why the heart is not working or whether a valve is failing or whether there is rubbish built up in the arteries. If I sketch what the problem is, it is suddenly much clearer for patients to understand. I let the patients take them away so they can ponder on it at home and come back with questions if need be. I might not be the best drawer but if you can't do that, there are so many illustrations and little films on YouTube to show your patients.

I think that doctors who do not pay enough attention to their communication skills should be retrained, including those doctors who don't listen to their patients. We regularly see women who are so-called "depressive" or "hysterical", or according to a previous doctor they saw—have problems with menopause, stress, hyperventilation, or other complaints which are "between the ears", but then after an investigation we find that they have cardiac arrhythmias! Compliancy of the patient with treatment starts with the doctor who puts in time to listen to his patient. He must explain everything as best he can, and in this way, transform a passive patient who is afraid to change, into a partner that is in charge of his own health. That is the reason why during this COVID crisis we decided to write this book—to help our patients and be a partner in their road to stay healthy.

ACKNOWLEDGMENTS

This book has been written with Your Heart in mind. But one does not write it all by oneself. The years of training in Medicine and Cardiology in particular, the experience I have received in helping and treating patients—it's all in here.

Therefore, a big THANK YOU to all our patients who helped to make us better partners in health care. A very special thanks to my friend and mentor, Professor Pedro Brugada, whose original idea it was to write a book like this for his patients together with journalist Marc Geenen who kindly gave me permission to do the same for mine. Mrs Karen Peradon-Alaga from Red Feather Publishing was the bright light during the Covid-19 darkness as she expertly guided me through the publishing process. Karen did a great job in editing, making the book 'readable'! I am in debt to my colleagues at Western Cardiology in Perth, Western Australia for supporting me and their willingness to expertly look after my patients when I was 'not around'. As mentioned, good patient care is a team effort and without the great help of my personal assistants Anita Waters and Rebecca Cocker... you, the patient, know what I mean! Without the expert typing skills of Tracy Howard, there would not have been a book within 9 months! And it was Jack Bendat, who kept pushing me each time to finish this book before the next basketball season! Thank you all.

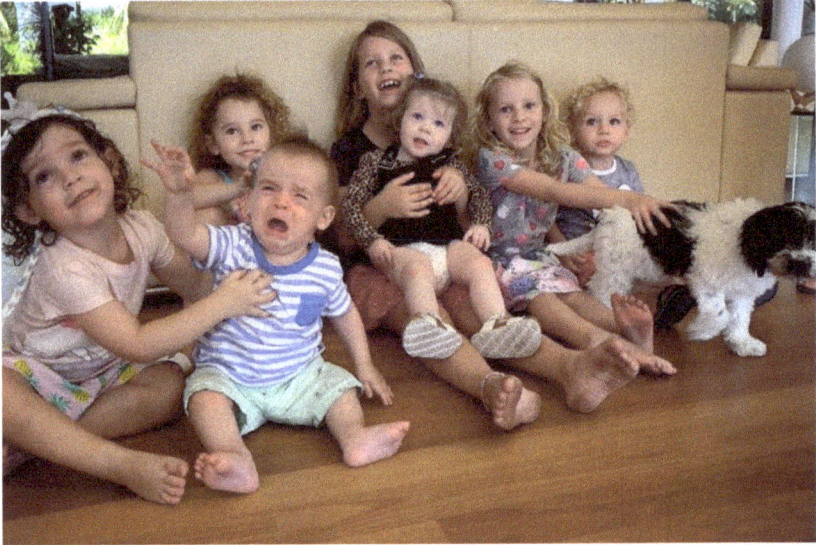

11

"Your Heart Maintenance" is dedicated to our seven grandkids: Ayla May, Jeanette, Simone, Sanne, Sebastian, Olivia and Van. And to my wife Marie-Louise, whose unwavering love and support keeps my Heart going.

Always.